Advances in Orbital, Oculoplastic and Lacrimal Surgery

Advances in Orbital, Oculoplastic and Lacrimal Surgery

Guest Editors

Kelvin Kam-Lung Chong
Renbing Jia

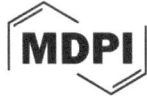

Basel • Beijing • Wuhan • Barcelona • Belgrade • Novi Sad • Cluj • Manchester

Guest Editors

Kelvin Kam-Lung Chong
Department of
Ophthalmology and Visual
Sciences
Faculty of Medicine
The Chinese University of
Hong Kong
Hong Kong
China

Renbing Jia
Department of
Ophthalmology
Ninth People's Hospital
Shanghai Jiao Tong
University School of Medicine
Shanghai
China

Editorial Office
MDPI AG
Grosspeteranlage 5
4052 Basel, Switzerland

This is a reprint of the Special Issue, published open access by the journal *Journal of Clinical Medicine* (ISSN 2077-0383), freely accessible at: https://www.mdpi.com/journal/jcm/special_issues/42Z6934OG3.

For citation purposes, cite each article independently as indicated on the article page online and as indicated below:

Lastname, A.A.; Lastname, B.B. Article Title. *Journal Name* **Year**, *Volume Number*, Page Range.

ISBN 978-3-7258-3155-5 (Hbk)
ISBN 978-3-7258-3156-2 (PDF)
https://doi.org/10.3390/books978-3-7258-3156-2

© 2025 by the authors. Articles in this book are Open Access and distributed under the Creative Commons Attribution (CC BY) license. The book as a whole is distributed by MDPI under the terms and conditions of the Creative Commons Attribution-NonCommercial-NoDerivs (CC BY-NC-ND) license (https://creativecommons.org/licenses/by-nc-nd/4.0/).

Contents

Karim Al-Ghazzawi, Inga Neumann, Mareile Knetsch, Ying Chen, Benjamin Wilde, Nikolaos E. Bechrakis, et al.
Treatment Outcomes of Patients with Orbital Inflammatory Diseases: Should Steroids Still Be the First Choice?
Reprinted from: *J. Clin. Med.* **2024**, *13*, 3998, https://doi.org/10.3390/jcm13143998 1

Steffani Krista Someda, Hidetaka Miyazaki, Hirohiko Kakizaki and Yasuhiro Takahashi
Clinical Significance of the Inferomedial Orbital Strut in Orbital Blowout Fractures: Incidence of Symptomatic Diplopia in a Fractured vs. Intact Strut
Reprinted from: *J. Clin. Med.* **2024**, *13*, 3682, https://doi.org/10.3390/jcm13133682 13

Seong Eun Lee, Hyung Bin Lim, Seungjun Oh, Kibum Lee and Sung Bok Lee
Effects of Topical Anti-Glaucoma Medications on Outcomes of Endoscopic Dacryocystorhinostomy: Comparison with Age- and Sex-Matched Controls
Reprinted from: *J. Clin. Med.* **2024**, *13*, 634, https://doi.org/10.3390/jcm13020634 22

Doah Kim and Helen Lew
Comparison of Outcomes of Silicone Tube Intubation with or without Dacryoendoscopy for the Treatment of Congenital Nasolacrimal Duct Obstruction
Reprinted from: *J. Clin. Med.* **2023**, *12*, 7370, https://doi.org/10.3390/jcm12237370 33

Yoshiki Ueta, Yuji Watanabe, Ryoma Kamada and Nobuya Tanaka
Assessment of Office-Based Probing with Dacryoendoscopy for Treatment of Congenital Nasolacrimal Duct Obstruction: A Retrospective Study
Reprinted from: *J. Clin. Med.* **2023**, *12*, 7048, https://doi.org/10.3390/jcm12227048 41

Steffani Krista Someda, Naomi Umezawa, Aric Vaidya, Hirohiko Kakizaki and Yasuhiro Takahashi
Surgical Outcomes of Bilateral Inferior Rectus Muscle Recession for Restrictive Strabismus Secondary to Thyroid Eye Disease
Reprinted from: *J. Clin. Med.* **2023**, *12*, 6876, https://doi.org/10.3390/jcm12216876 49

Yuri Kim and Helen Lew
Recovery of the Ratio of Closure Time during Blink Time in Lacrimal Passage Intubation
Reprinted from: *J. Clin. Med.* **2023**, *12*, 3631, https://doi.org/10.3390/jcm12113631 62

Xulin Liao, Kenneth Ka Hei Lai, Fatema Mohamed Ali Abdulla Aljufairi, Wanxue Chen, Zhichao Hu, Hanson Yiu Man Wong, et al.
Ocular Surface Changes in Treatment-Naive Thyroid Eye Disease
Reprinted from: *J. Clin. Med.* **2023**, *12*, 3066, https://doi.org/10.3390/jcm12093066 72

Xulin Liao, Fatema Mohamed Ali Abdulla Aljufairi, Kenneth Ka Hei Lai, Karen Kar Wun Chan, Ruofan Jia, Wanxue Chen, et al.
Clinical Significance of Corneal Striae in Thyroid Associated Orbitopathy
Reprinted from: *J. Clin. Med.* **2023**, *12*, 2284, https://doi.org/10.3390/jcm12062284 80

Umberto Committeri, Antonio Arena, Emanuele Carraturo, Martina Austoni, Cristiana Germano, Giovanni Salzano, et al.
Incidence of Orbital Side Effects in Zygomaticomaxillary Complex and Isolated Orbital Walls Fractures: A Retrospective Study in South Italy and a Brief Review of the Literature
Reprinted from: *J. Clin. Med.* **2023**, *12*, 845, https://doi.org/10.3390/jcm12030845 90

Pei-Yuan Su, Jia-Kang Wang and Shu-Wen Chang
Computed Tomography Morphology of Affected versus Unaffected Sides in Patients with Unilateral Primary Acquired Nasolacrimal Duct Obstruction
Reprinted from: *J. Clin. Med.* **2023**, *12*, 340, https://doi.org/10.3390/jcm12010340 . . . . **99**

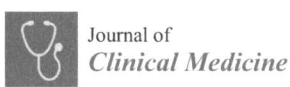

Article

Treatment Outcomes of Patients with Orbital Inflammatory Diseases: Should Steroids Still Be the First Choice?

Karim Al-Ghazzawi [1,*], Inga Neumann [1], Mareile Knetsch [1], Ying Chen [1], Benjamin Wilde [2], Nikolaos E. Bechrakis [1], Anja Eckstein [1,†] and Michael Oeverhaus [1,*,†]

[1] Department of Ophthalmology, University Hospital Essen, 45147 Essen, Germany
[2] Department of Nephrology, University Hospital Essen, 45147 Essen, Germany
* Correspondence: karim.al-ghazzawi@uk-essen.de (K.A.-G.); m.oeverhaus@web.de (M.O.)
† These authors contributed equally to the work.

Abstract: Objective: To clarify the therapy response in orbital inflammatory diseases (OID), we analyzed the treatment effects of steroid therapy, the use of disease-modifying antirheumatic drugs (DMARDS), and biologicals in our tertiary referral center cohort. **Methods**: We collected the clinical and demographic data of all patients treated for non-specific orbital inflammation (NSOI) (*n* = 111) and IgG4-ROD (*n* = 13), respectively at our center from 2008 to 2020 and analyzed them with descriptive statistics. NSOI were sub-grouped according to the location into either idiopathic dacryoadenitis (DAs) (*n* = 78) or typical idiopathic orbital myositis (*n* = 32). **Results**: Mean age at first clinical manifestation was significantly different between subgroups (IOI: 49.5 ± 18, IgG4-ROD: 63.2 ± 14, *p* = 0.0171). Among all examined OID, 63 patients (50%) achieved full remission (FR) with corticosteroids (NSOI 53%/IgG4-ROD 31%). In contrast, classic myositis showed a significantly higher response (76%). Disease-modifying drugs (DMARDS) for myositis accomplished only 33% FR (NSOI 57%) and 66% did not respond sufficiently (NSOI 43%). The biologic agent (Rituximab) was significantly more efficient: 19 of 23 patients (82%) achieved full remission and only 4 (17%) did not respond fully and needed orbital irradiation or orbital decompressive surgery.

Keywords: NSOI; IgG4-ROD; OID; inflammation; biologicals; steroids; myositis; dacryoadenitis; lacrimal gland

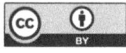

Citation: Al-Ghazzawi, K.; Neumann, I.; Knetsch, M.; Chen, Y.; Wilde, B.; Bechrakis, N.E.; Eckstein, A.; Oeverhaus, M. Treatment Outcomes of Patients with Orbital Inflammatory Diseases: Should Steroids Still Be the First Choice? *J. Clin. Med.* **2024**, *13*, 3998. https://doi.org/10.3390/jcm13143998

Academic Editor: Brent Siesky

Received: 6 May 2024
Revised: 8 June 2024
Accepted: 29 June 2024
Published: 9 July 2024

Copyright: © 2024 by the authors. Licensee MDPI, Basel, Switzerland. This article is an open access article distributed under the terms and conditions of the Creative Commons Attribution (CC BY) license (https://creativecommons.org/licenses/by/4.0/).

1. Introduction

Orbital inflammatory diseases (OID) encompass a wide range of pathologies, including isolated diseases such as IgG4-related orbital disease (IgG4-ROD), non-specific orbital inflammation (NSOI, formerly orbital pseudotumor), and manifestations of systemic diseases such as the most common thyroid eye disease (TED), granulomatosis with polyangiitis (GPA), Sjögren syndrome (SjS), and sarcoidosis [1–4], among others. They can affect any tissue of the orbit focally or diffusely, with presentations ranging from abrupt to insidious onset. Symptoms vary depending on the affected tissues, but typically include pain, proptosis, periorbital edema and erythema, impaired motility, and consequently diplopia in most cases, and sometimes decreased visual acuity [1,3,5]. Differential diagnosis includes isolated and systemic autoimmune diseases, lymphoproliferative diseases, and infectious diseases [6,7]. Therefore, an extensive laboratory and imaging workup, including autoimmune markers, is recommended [1,8,9]. Some specific autoimmune conditions can be identified in this way (TED, GPA, classical ocular myositis). However, in all other cases, diagnosis relies mostly on histopathological findings after orbital biopsy [10]. In the future, advances in MRI technology and AI-based diagnostics might overcome this hurdle [11]. Despite all advances, NSOI remains an exclusion diagnosis [1]. Classical myositis is usually treated with corticosteroids without performing a biopsy first [1,12]. Dose regimens vary due to the lack of an international or European guideline (20–80 mg/day or 1 mg/kg body weight per day, tapered) [9]. Typical myositis subsides under treatment within 2–3 days.

In contrast, treatment of NSOI and IgG4-ROD is challenging. Some patients respond very well to (a) systemic steroid therapy, while others need multiple cycles and (b) additional immunosuppressive agents (DMARDs) as maintenance therapy to prevent relapses and achieve a stable state; however, if still not responsive to therapy (c) biologicals can be applied usually in cases with recalcitrant nonspecific orbital inflammation. Some even require (d) irradiation or debulking surgery [1,13]. Patients might be spared unnecessary recurrences if treated early with effective immunosuppressive treatments, but currently, predictive factors are still missing [14–16]. Immunosuppressive Agents (DMARDs) are beneficial for patients with non-responsiveness or recurrence post-corticosteroid therapy: Methotrexate; Cyclosporin-A; Mycophenolate mofetil (MMF); Cyclophosphamide, Sulfasalazine, and Azathioprine (AZA) [17,18]. Since IgG4-ROD shows a high relapse rate of about 50% [19,20], MTX, AZA, MMF, Infliximab, Cyclophosphamide, and Rituximab (RTX) should be considered early for effective treatment [21]. Biologicals such as RTX seem to be most effective for IgG4-ROD, with up to 94% remission in a recent review [22]. Comparable results have also been achieved in NSOI patients [23]. Alternatively, MTX, MMF, tocilizumab, infliximab, and adalimumab can be used for NSOI [1,24]. Unfortunately, only a few small randomized controlled trials are available for NSOI and IgG4-ROD. Thus, most treatments are 'off-label' and financial coverage needs to be applied for with health insurance companies. Only GPA patients benefit from the approval of the EMA for RTX in 2013, and long-term data are available [25]. Therefore, we aimed to analyze our tertiary referral center cohort of patients with NSOI and IgG4-ROD for treatment effects in terms of stable disease and possible clinical predictors for the effectiveness of the different therapeutic modalities.

2. Patients and Methods

2.1. Study Population

We identified 127 patients with typical clinical course and certain diagnoses for NSOI ($n = 114$), and IgG4-ROD ($n = 13$) from our patient database comprised of patient records between 2008 and 2020. NSOI were sub-grouped into either typical idiopathic dacryoadenitis (idiopathic DAs) ($n = 78$) or idiopathic orbital myositis ($n = 32$). The study was performed under adherence to the ethical foundations of the Declaration of Helsinki and was approved by the Ethics Commission of the University of Essen (11-4822-B0). Diagnosis of NSOI and IgG4-ROD were based on clinical, flow cytometric, and histological (including immunostaining) examinations. IgG4-ROD was diagnosed in accordance with the published 2020 revised comprehensive diagnostic (RCD) criteria [26]. Briefly, IgG4-ROD was diagnosed in the presence of (1) one or more organs showing diffuse or localized swelling or a mass or nodule characteristic of IgG4-RD. In single-organ involvement, lymph node swelling is omitted. (2) Serum IgG4 levels greater than 135 mg/dL. (3) Positivity for two of the following three criteria: (a) dense lymphocyte and plasma cell infiltration with fibrosis; (b) ratio of IgG4-positive plasma cells/IgG-positive cells greater than 40% and the number of IgG4-positive plasma cells greater than 10 per high-powered field; and (c) typical tissue fibrosis, particularly storiform fibrosis, or obliterative phlebitis.

Patients who fulfilled all 3 criteria were considered as definitive IgG4-RD. Patients with (1) and (2) or (1) and (3) were regarded as definitive IgG4-RD if they fulfill the organ-specific criteria for IgG4-RD. Cases that did not meet the inclusion criteria or had incomplete datasets (loss to follow-up) were excluded.

2.2. Statistical Evaluation

To analyze metric data, median values ($\tilde{x}$) and range or mean and standard deviation (SD) were computed. A student's t-test (two-tailed) was used to assess differences between groups if the D'Agostino–Pearson omnibus normality test indicated normal distribution; otherwise, the Mann–Whitney Test was used. Fisher's exact test was used to examine group distributions of binary variables. For the comparison of ordinal variables and factors with more than two groups, either the Kruskal–Wallis test (non-parametric) or ANOVA (parametric) were used to detect group differences. All calculations were performed with SPSS (IBM SPSS Statistics, Chicago, IL, USA, Version 22.0.0,) and Graph Pad Prism (Prism 9 for Windows, Software Inc., San Diego, CA, USA, Version 9.0.0). *p*-values are given descriptively without α-adjustment for multiple testing.

2.3. Clinical Data Collection

General information was collected from the medical records database at baseline and follow-up examinations, including age, gender, affected eye, symptoms, previous history (including previous glucocorticoid therapy prior to referral), clinical manifestations, serum blood results, imaging findings, immunohistochemical indicators, and given treatments. Pathological diagnosis was confirmed by a minimum of two pathologists. If histopathological diagnosis was uncertain a tertiary referral pathologist of an independent center was consulted.

2.4. Imaging and Biopsy

Prior to biopsy, all patients received an orbital imaging modality. Magnetic resonance imaging (MRI) and/or computed tomography (CT), were obtained and evaluated by neuroradiologists. A biopsy of the lesions was performed when it was considered necessary to confirm the diagnosis. If extra-ophthalmic manifestation was suspected, systemic imaging was performed.

2.5. Treatment Protocol

2.5.1. Glucocorticosteroids (GC)

The GC-tapering regimen varied. Depending on the severity of the NSOI ranging GC pulse was started with a dose between 0.75 mg prednisolone/Kg Bodyweight and 1.5 mg prednisolone/Kg Bodyweight and tapered off slowly over weeks.

2.5.2. DMARDs

Therapy was only commenced after ruling out contraindications e.g., lymphopenia, systemic severe infections, latent tuberculosis (TBC), uncontrolled cardiac disease, and pregnancy. In addition, the vaccination status was optimized.

Mycophenolate Mofetil

Mycophenolate Mofetil was given at a dose of 2×360 mg per day, orally. The recommendation was given for separate doses per day taken with meals to improve gastrointestinal tolerance. Mycophenolate leads to a relatively selective inhibition of DNA replication in T- and B-cells.

Methotrexate

Methotrexate was initiated at the same time as Corticosteroids at a dose of 15–20 mg per week, orally or preferably subcutaneously, along with folic acid supplementation. The drug inhibits dihydrofolate reductase and suppresses both B- and T-cells.

Cyclophosphamide

Cyclophosphamide was given at a dose of 15 mg/kg as pulse therapy over two to four cycles or as an oral continuous therapy at 2 mg/kg/d. Its cytotoxic effect is mainly due to cross-linking of DNA strands (alkylating agent), therefore inhibiting protein synthesis.

Cyclosporin A

Cyclosporin A was given was given to patients at a starting dose of 4 mg/kg/day and tapered to 2 mg/kg/day. The drug suppresses lymphocyte-mediated responses, inhibits T cells, and decreases the production of IL-1 and IL-2.

Azathioprine

Azathioprine was given was given to patients in a dose of 2–3 mg/kg/day. It is an antagonist of purines, resulting in the inhibition of DNA, RNA, and protein synthesis.

Sulfasalazine

Sulfasalazine exerts its anti-inflammatory effects through multiple mechanisms. Proposed mechanisms of action: inhibition of the transcription factor nuclear factor kappa-B (NF-kB), which leads to the suppression of NF-kB responsive pro-inflammatory genes, including TNF-α. Additionally, sulfasalazine induces caspase 8-induced apoptosis in macrophages, thereby inhibiting TNF-α expression.

2.5.3. Biologicals

Rituximab (CD-20 Inhibitor)

RTX is a monoclonal antibody that targets the CD20 antigen found on the surface of B cells. The working principle of rituximab involves: 1. Depletion of B Cells: Rituximab binds to the CD20 antigen on the surface of B cells, leading to the destruction of these cells. 2. Modulation of Immune Response: By targeting B cells, rituximab can modulate the immune response. 3. Impact on Autoimmune Diseases: In autoimmune diseases, B-cells play a role in the production of autoantibodies and the presentation of autoantigens. Rituximab's ability to deplete B cells can help in reducing autoantibody levels and suppressing the autoimmune response. It was given as an off-label treatment to patients. Rituximab was given as 2 intravenous doses of (500 mg to 1 g) 2 weeks apart in addition to standard treatment.

Treatment Outcome

We defined therapy response to corticosteroids as follows:
- Full Remission: Patients who responded to corticosteroids over a maximum of two courses with a remission of clinical symptoms and pain without a recurrence over the observed time of this study;
- Partial Remission: Patients that responded initially to corticosteroids with a remission of clinical symptoms, but needed a second immunosuppressive agent (DMARDs or Biologicals) due to incomplete response recurrence dosage >10 mg.

We defined therapy response to steroids in combination with DMARDS as follows:
- Full Remission: Patients that responded to a combination of corticosteroids (maximum 7.5 mg/day) with DMARDS, without a recurrence over the observed time of this study;
- Partial Remission: Patients that responded initially to a combination of higher-dosed corticosteroids with DMARDS with a remission of clinical symptoms but needed treatment with Biologicals due to incomplete response or recurrence of disease with steroids >10 mg.

We defined therapy response to biologicals as follows:
- Full Remission: Patients that responded to a combination of corticosteroids (maximum 7.5 mg/day) with biologicals without a recurrence over the observed time of this study;
- Partial Remission: Patients that did not respond sufficiently to treatment with biologicals and corticosteroids (>7.5 mg/day).

3. Results

3.1. Study Population and Characteristics of OID

The 124 patients ranged in age from 9 to 91 years (mean 51.9 years); 55 were male, and 69 were female. Observed age as well as sex predilection was different between observed entities, $p = 0.04$ and $p = 0.03$, respectively (Table 1). The left eye was affected in 55 patients, the right eye in 58 patients, and both eyes in 11 patients. In 78 out of 127 (62%) cases, a biopsy was performed in our institution to confirm the diagnosis in addition to clinical presentation. Forty cases were treated without a biopsy. The remaining 14 patients had external biopsies, a clear diagnosis due to a diagnosed systemic disease, or refused to undergo surgery due to comorbidities. Idiopathic DAs were more likely to be biopsied $p < 0.0001$ (Table 1).

Table 1. Population characteristics in our index population stratified for each disease entity and subtype of disease.

	All OIDs	Myositis	Idiopathic DA $n = 79$	IgG4-ROD $n = 13$	p
Age	51.9 ± 17.76	49.26 ± 16.08	49.67 ± 18.7	63 ± 13.83	0.0492 [a]
Unilateral manifestation	113 (91.2%)	28	72	13	0.42 [b]
Male sex	55 (44.3%)	12	38	5	0.0392 [b]
Biopsy	84 (67.74%)	7	64	13	0.0001 [b]

Unless otherwise stated, data are means ± SD or are proportions (%) or counts [a]: Welch ANOVA test. [b]: Kruskal–Wallis test.

The median duration of time between first clinical presentation and biopsy was 6.9 ± 5 months. The patients presented with a range of signs and symptoms. A swelling/mass was the most common presentation other than proptosis, pain, extraocular muscle restriction, diplopia, ptosis, and decreased vision (Table 2).

Table 2. Clinical symptoms present in our index population stratified for each disease entity and subtype of disease.

Entity	Eyelid Swelling	Proptosis	Limited Eye Movement	Visual Loss	Diplopia	Orbital Pain
Myositis $n = 32$	23 (72%)	8 (25%)	15 (47%)	8 (25%)	13 (41%)	26 (81%)
idiopathic DAs $n = 79$	53 (67%)	53 (67%)	44 (56%)	31 (39%)	50 (63%)	64 (81%)
IgG4-ROD $n = 13$	8 (62%)	8 (62)	7 (54%)	8 (62%)	5 (38%)	6 (46%)

3.2. Therapy Response

3.2.1. Classical Myositis

Response to corticosteroids was very high in classical myositis when compared to the overall study population (Figure 1): Most patients (78%) achieved remission after a maximum of two corticosteroid courses (Table 3). Two patients achieved remission after GC + DMARDS, but four patients needed treatment with RTX. All four unresponsive cases to DMARDs were biopsied to rule out malignancies before therapy with RTX. Despite all treatments, 2/32 patients only responded partially and were therefore subjected to radiation therapy. One patient who responded initially while being treated with RTX, but who diseased before the remission of clinical symptoms could be achieved, was counted as partial remission.

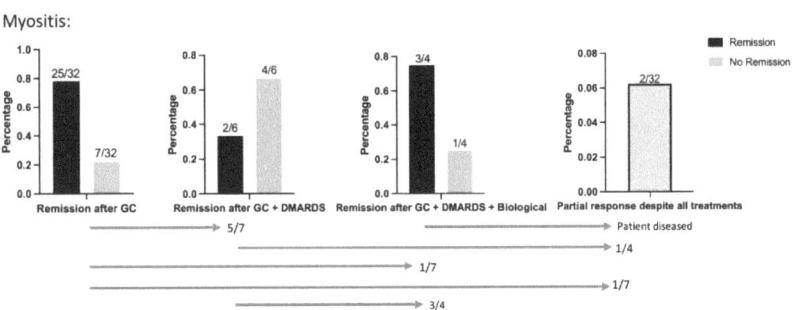

Figure 1. Treatment efficacy in Myositis cases. Blue bars show patient flow between cohorts; 25/32 achieved remission after a maximum of two corticosteroid courses, 8/25 (32%) being male patients. Five patients were subjected to GC + DMARDs, of whom two patients achieved remission. Four patients treated with GC + DMARDs needed treatment with RTX to achieve remission.

Table 3. Clinical remission after treatment in our index population stratified for each disease entity and subtype of treatment. Stated data are proportions (%). [a]: Fisher's exact test in glucocorticoids vs. group.

	All	Remission after Treatment	No Remission	p
Myositis	32	30	2	
Glucocorticoids	32	(78%) 25	(22%) 7	
DMARDs	6	(33.3%) 2	(66.7%) 4	0.046 [a]
Biologicals	4	(75%) 3	(25%) 1	1 [a]
Idiopathic DAs	78	61	17	
Glucocorticoids	78	(42%) 33	(58%) 43	
DMARDs	24	(62.5%) 15	(37.5%) 9	0.3571 [a]
Biologicals	12	(92%) 11	(8%) 1	0.0035 [a]
IgG4-ROD	13	10	3	
Glucocorticoids	13	(30%) 4	(70%) 9	
DMARDs	1	(100%) 1	0	0.357 [a]
Biologicals	7	(71%) 5	(19%) 2	0.15 [a]

3.2.2. Treatment Efficacy in Dacryoadenitis

After treatment with corticosteroids, inactive disease was achieved in 42% of 78 patients with DA (Figure 2). GC + DMARDS (Cyclophosphamides, Azathioprine, MTX, and Cyclosporin A) were applied in 24/78 cases. Of these, 63% of patients achieved inactive disease. MTX (15 mg/week subcutaneous; in single cases 20 mg/week for 4–40 months) was used as monotherapy in 14/24 cases. Both Cyclophosphamide (1 g/4-courses) and Mycophenolate monotherapy (350–750 mg/day for 6–36 months) were noted in 2/24 cases (1 g over 2–3 courses/(750 mg/day)). Azathioprine (150 mg–200 mg/day for 4 months) and Cyclosporin (4–2 mg/kg bodyweight/day for 2 months) were used in one case, respectively. The therapy regimen MTX + Azathioprine (15–20 mg/weekly + 150–200 mg/day for 4–40 months), MTX + MMF (20 mg/day + 500 mg/day for 24 months), or MTX + Sulfasalazine (20 mg/day + 500 mg/day for 36 months) was noted in 6/24 cases. Insufficient response to DMARDs and therapeutic switch to a biological (Rituximab) was necessary in 6/24 cases. Complete therapeutic switch to biologicals (Rituximab) due to insufficient response to Corticosteroids while organ-threatening orbital disease was observed was necessary in 7.6% (6/78) of cases. Biologicals (Rituximab) were applied in 12 DA patients. Here, full remission was achieved in 91% (11/12), of which one patient showed only partial response despite all treatments. Altogether 17/78 (24%) patients responded only partially despite all treatments. Here, (10/17) were treated with radiation therapy of which 7 received additional surgical decompression. In all 14/17 patients were surgically decompressed due to organ-threatening behavior of the orbital mass. Supplemental Figure S1 demonstrates the time of relapse under DMARD vs. GC therapy. In patients with recurrent DAs, the interval between the Inflammatory episode and the recurrence under therapy was shorter in GC (86% relapse-free survival in DMARDs vs. 64% relapse-free survival in GC after 2 months of treatment).

3.2.3. IgG4-ROD

The initial response to corticosteroids was 100%. However, 69% of patients relapsed when corticosteroids were tapered (prednisolone 7.5 mg, Figure 3). One relapsed patient received DMARDS (Mycophenolate 750 mg for 3 years) monotherapy, which achieved remission. Rituximab was given to the other seven relapsed patients and achieved remission in 71%. Decompressive surgery was necessary in three patients due to insufficient response despite all treatments.

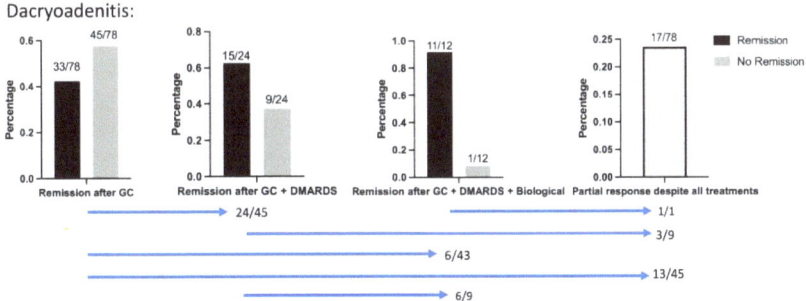

Figure 2. Definitive therapy in the examined DAs. GC achieved remission in 42%, and DMARDS (Cyclophosphamid, Azathioprin, MTX, or Cyclosporin A) achieved remission in 62.5%. Remission was achieved with Rituximab in 91%. Blue bars show patient flow between cohorts; Despite all treatments, 19/78 patients could not achieve remission (24%). A biopsy to rule out malignancies (e.g., Lymphoma) was performed in all patients treated with DMARDs, Biologicals, as well as nonresponsive recalcitrant DAs. In total, 64/79 DAs were biopsied.

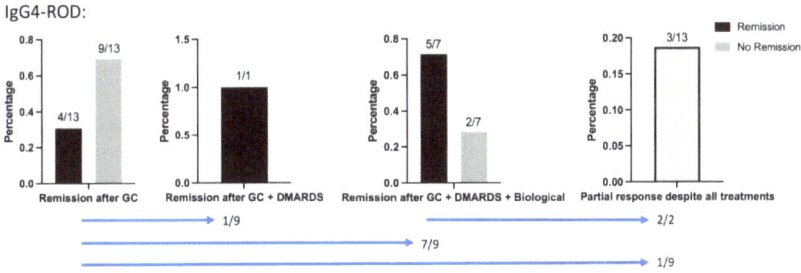

Figure 3. Response to all therapies in examined IgG4-ROD cases. Blue bars show patient flow between cohorts; 9/13 patients relapsed when corticosteroids were tapered and were therefore subjected to other therapies. One relapsed patient received DMARDS monotherapy, which achieved remission. Rituximab was given to the other seven relapsed patients and achieved remission in 5/7 cases; 3/13 patients were subjected to decompressive surgery in organ-threatening disease manifestations.

4. Discussion

The results of this retrospective analysis of patient data from 124 patients with NSOI (DA and Myositis) and IgG4 from our tertiary referral center showed significantly different treatment outcomes, depending on the disease entity and localization. Whereas orbital myositis mostly showed promising remission with GC monotherapy, idiopathic dacryoadenitis showed a much higher relapse rate and demanded second-line treatments, such as DMARDs and biologicals. Unlike other organ manifestations, which seem to respond well to GC monotherapy, our small group of isolated IgG4-ROD needed second-line therapies in two-thirds of the patients and even surgery to avoid dramatic consequences for the visual function.

4.1. Treatment of NSOI

First-line treatment for NSOI remains high-dose corticosteroids, tapered off slowly over months. Often the tapering is carried out too quickly, resulting in a "relapse", which is more an improper treatment of the orbital inflammation. GCs come with the perks of being affordable, easily accessible, and quite effective in addressing NSOIs. In patients that show positive responses to the drug, complaints, and especially pain start to diminish quickly.

4.1.1. Myositis

There are no well-designed, randomized controlled clinical trials for the treatment of myositis, and most publications are small, retrospective case studies. NSAIDs have been used in the past, though GCs are still first-line therapy, and currently colleagues have reported increased use of DMARDs (Supplemental Table S1 includes several publications with myositis cases). GCs were reported to be effective in 60–74% of cases. DMARDs (Azathioprine and MTX) have been reported effective in 60–80%, but have only been administered in a few cases (seven cases in total). Biologicals have been reported to be effective in irresponsive cases with multiple relapses. This was also true in our study cohort, which points out the positive effect of Biologicals (RTX) in relapsing myositis cases. In addition, the biological TNF-alpha (Infliximab) has been reported effective in chronic orbital myositis [27] with promising results (71% remission). However, due to small patient numbers, further studies of this agent for recurring orbital myositis cases are needed. To the best of our knowledge, our study is the first study with the largest patient cohort illustrating detailed therapy responses to each medication.

4.1.2. Dacryoadenitis

The observed response rate was quite low in GC monotherapy with only 42%. This is in accordance with previous literature reporting an estimate of 20% to 60% recurrence in patients with dacryoadenitis (Supplemental Table S2) [10,28,29]. Due to this low remission rate for idiopathic DAs, an additional immunosuppressive agent (DMARD) is recommended and therapeutic preparation (e.g., blood examination to rule out contraindications) should be performed very early [24,30]. The side-effect profile of long-term corticosteroids, includes adrenal insufficiency, cataract, osteoporosis, psychosis, diabetes, and gastrointestinal disorders and should not be underestimated [31]. Typical DMARD medication includes cyclosporine-A, methotrexate, cyclophosphamide, tacrolimus, azathioprine, and mycophenolate mofetil [32–34]. The patient number per specific DMARD was rather low, which is why further studies are needed to elucidate the response to the monotherapies. Methotrexate is the most used steroid-sparing immunomodulating agent for the management of orbital inflammation, most probably due to its low risk/benefit ratio. Side effects include fatigue, hair loss, gastrointestinal disturbance, and elevated liver enzymes [35]. Supplementing dietary folate and regular monitoring of liver enzymes are needed to minimize these adverse effects is recommended.

Monoclonal antibodies have now been highlighted as novel immunomodulating agents. These biologic drugs are highly specific and have proven to be superior to conventional immunosuppressive drugs regarding their efficacy and safety for specific indications in more common autoimmune diseases. We analyzed 12 cases with Rituximab and could show its effectiveness as a second-line treatment (90% remission). This is in line with previously published results [14,23]. The excellent response compared to other DMARDs should lead to an early consideration of RTX. Recurring autoantibodies in patients who present with NSOI, in combination with its association with immunological inflammatory disorders, e.g., Crohn's disease, rheumatoid arthritis, diabetes mellitus, systemic lupus erythematosus, hints at an underlying autoimmune process [36]. Some authors even suggest RTX as first-line therapy in idiopathic DAs, since patients often show complete remission after one cycle, preventing fibrosis in adipose tissue and complicated courses [16,23]. TNF-alpha blockers have been reported effective in the treatment of irresponsive, relapsing NSOI [37]. Our study also points out the efficacy of success over time when observing relapse-free survival (Supplemental Figure S1). Altogether, both therapy success and observed relapse-free survival are proving a more efficient therapy in DMARDs and biologicals compared to GC monotherapy. Relapsing drug-resistant cases were observed in 17 cases for our examined DA cohort. For these patients, only radiation and surgery remain, especially in sight-threatening manifestations. Radiation has historically been considered an effective alternative in recalcitrant or recurrent NSOIs [38]. Surgery has been proposed to be effective in infiltrative fibrosing non-responsive NSOIs [39]. Further studies are needed to affirm the theory that some patients with NSOIs might profit from early therapy with biologicals, especially before fibrosis within the adipose tissue occurs. Improved orbital imaging and molecular profiling of biopsies might be crucial to determine which patients can profit from early biologicals [7].

4.2. Treatment of IgG4-ROD

Patients with IgG4-related disease (IgG-RD) typically respond well at first to corticosteroids, especially in the early phases of the disease [40]. Serum IgG4 levels, lymphocytic infiltration, as well as clinical symptoms such as organ enlargement, pain, or diplopia usually improve within the first weeks. In an international consensus, GC is therefore recommended as a first-line induction treatment [41]. A small minority of relapsing patients, however, do need a second immunosuppressive agent [42]. In patients with orbital manifestation, this seems to be different at least in our cohort. In our cohort, 38% of patients showed remission with only GC. However, the majority (62%) relapsed when corticosteroids were tapered. This is why it is recommended to consider DMARDs early on in IgG4-ROD similar to idiopathic DAs [21]. The relapsed patients of our cohort were either treated with DMARDs, debulking surgery, or Rituximab. The last achieved remission in 71% of cases, compared to only 25% in DMARDs. This is a bit lower compared to other studies analyzing the effects of RTX (94%) but could be rather explained by the small number of patients [22]. All observed patients who achieved remission showed a stable remission after one or two courses of RTX without late recurrences that demanded additional immunosuppressive agents. This might indicate that IgG4-ROD patients should be evaluated early on in case of a relapse after GCs for RTX treatment to avoid a chronic treatment with DMARDs. Further studies are needed to confirm the observed long-term effect of RTX on IgG4-ROD after 1–2 courses.

4.3. Limitations

The interpretation of our results is limited by its retrospective design and the typical. However, due to the rather high amount of patients considering the low incidence of the diseases, we think that our data are very useful to improve OID therapy. Future studies should be planned in a multicentric prospective design to further elucidate this matter. Ideally, they should include elaborate imaging protocols and molecular testing of the diseased patients.

5. Conclusions

Our single-center retrospective analysis emphasized the difficulty of treating patients with OIDs. Corticosteroids were confirmed as a viable option for idiopathic orbital myositis and induction therapy for patients with more severe NSOI and IgG4-ROD; however, the common relapses in these patients demonstrate the need for an early alternative immunosuppressive therapy. DMARDs are shown to be only partially effective. RTX, on the other hand, was, in our cohorts, the most effective second-line treatment and should be considered as an early second-line option, especially due to the excellent long-term results.

Supplementary Materials: The following supporting information can be downloaded at: https://www.mdpi.com/article/10.3390/jcm13143998/s1. Figure S1. Proportions of relapse free survival: CS vs. DMARDs in DAs. Table S1. Literature Summary of Patients reported with Orbital Myositis and treatment outcomes. Table S2. Literature Summary of Patients reported with isolated Dacryoadenitis and treatment outcomes. References [43–49] are cited in the Supplementary Materials.

Author Contributions: Data curation, K.A.-G., M.K. and B.W.; formal analysis, K.A.-G., Y.C., A.E. and M.O.; funding acquisition, A.E. and M.O.; investigation, K.A.-G., I.N., M.K., Y.C., A.E. and M.O.; methodology, K.A.-G., N.E.B., A.E. and M.O.; project administration, A.E.; resources, K.A.-G., I.N., M.K., Y.C., B.W. and N.E.B.; supervision, N.E.B., A.E. and M.O.; validation, K.A.-G., A.E. and M.O.; visualization, K.A.-G.; writing—original draft, K.A.-G. and M.O.; writing—review and editing, K.A.-G., I.N., B.W. and M.O. All authors have read and agreed to the published version of the manuscript.

Funding: This research received funding from the German Research Foundation and the University Hospital Essen (UMEA program, FU 356/12-2). We acknowledge support by the Open Access Publication Fund of the University of Duisburg-Essen.

Institutional Review Board Statement: The study was performed in adherence to the ethical foundations of the Declaration of Helsinki and was approved by the Ethics Commission of the University of Essen (11-4822-B0) on 13 October 2020.

Informed Consent Statement: Patient consent was waived due to the retrospective nature of this study by the Ethics Committee.

Data Availability Statement: The data that support the findings of this study are available from the corresponding author, M.O., upon reasonable request.

Conflicts of Interest: The authors state that there are no conflicts of interest. The funders had no role in the design of the study; in the collection, analyses, or interpretation of data; in the writing of the manuscript; or in the decision to publish the results.

References

1. Lee, M.J.; Planck, S.R.; Choi, D.; Harrington, C.A.; Wilson, D.J.; Dailey, R.A.; Ng, J.D.; Steele, E.A.; Hamilton, B.E.; Khwarg, S.I.; et al. Non-specific orbital inflammation: Current understanding and unmet needs. *Prog. Retin. Eye Res.* **2021**, *81*, 100885. [CrossRef]
2. Gunalp, I.; Gunduz, K.; Yazar, Z. Idiopathic orbital inflammatory disease. *Acta Ophthalmol. Scand.* **1996**, *74*, 191–193. [CrossRef]
3. Swamy, B.N.; McCluskey, P.; Nemet, A.; Crouch, R.; Martin, P.; Benger, R.; Ghabriel, R.; Wakefield, D. Idiopathic orbital inflammatory syndrome: Clinical features and treatment outcomes. *Br. J. Ophthalmol.* **2007**, *91*, 1667–1670. [CrossRef]
4. Wallace, Z.S.; Deshpande, V.; Stone, J.H. Ophthalmic manifestations of IgG4-related disease: Single-center experience and literature review. *Semin. Arthritis Rheum.* **2014**, *43*, 806–817. [CrossRef]
5. Harris, G.J. Idiopathic orbital inflammation: A pathogenetic construct and treatment strategy: The 2005 ASOPRS Foundation Lecture. *Ophthalmic Plast Reconstr. Surg.* **2006**, *22*, 79–86. [CrossRef]
6. Klingenstein, A.; Hintschich, C. Specific inflammations of the orbit. *Ophthalmologe* **2021**, *118*, 794–800. [CrossRef]
7. Al-Ghazzawi, K.; Mairinger, F.D.; Pfortner, R.; Horstmann, M.; Bechrakis, N.; Mohr, C.; Eckstein, A.; Oeverhaus, M. Novel Insights into Pathophysiology of Orbital Inflammatory Diseases and Progression to Orbital Lymphoma by Pathway Enrichment Analysis. *Life* **2022**, *12*, 1660. [CrossRef]
8. Tsukikawa, M.; Lally, S.E.; Shields, C.L.; Eagle, R.C., Jr.; Ellis, F.J.; Wasserman, B.N. Idiopathic Orbital Pseudotumor Preceding Systemic Inflammatory Disease in Children. *J. Pediatr. Ophthalmol. Strabismus* **2019**, *56*, 373–377. [CrossRef]
9. Jacobs, D.; Galetta, S. Diagnosis and management of orbital pseudotumor. *Curr. Opin. Ophthalmol.* **2002**, *13*, 347–351. [CrossRef]
10. Al-Ghazzawi, K.; Baum, S.H.; Pfortner, R.; Philipp, S.; Bechrakis, N.; Gortz, G.; Eckstein, A.; Mairinger, F.D.; Oeverhaus, M. Evaluation of Orbital Lymphoproliferative and Inflammatory Disorders by Gene Expression Analysis. *Int. J. Mol. Sci.* **2022**, *23*, 8609. [CrossRef]
11. Xie, X.; Yang, L.; Zhao, F.; Wang, D.; Zhang, H.; He, X.; Cao, X.; Yi, H.; He, X.; Hou, Y. A deep learning model combining multimodal radiomics, clinical and imaging features for differentiating ocular adnexal lymphoma from idiopathic orbital inflammation. *Eur. Radiol.* **2022**, *32*, 6922–6932. [CrossRef]
12. Lutt, J.R.; Lim, L.L.; Phal, P.M.; Rosenbaum, J.T. Orbital inflammatory disease. *Semin. Arthritis Rheum.* **2008**, *37*, 207–222. [CrossRef]
13. Chen, J.; Zhang, P.; Ye, H.; Xiao, W.; Chen, R.; Mao, Y.; Ai, S.; Liu, Z.; Tang, L.; Yang, H. Clinical features and outcomes of IgG4-related idiopathic orbital inflammatory disease: From a large southern China-based cohort. *Eye* **2021**, *35*, 1248–1255. [CrossRef]
14. Suhler, E.B.; Lim, L.L.; Beardsley, R.M.; Giles, T.R.; Pasadhika, S.; Lee, S.T.; de Saint Sardos, A.; Butler, N.J.; Smith, J.R.; Rosenbaum, J.T. Rituximab therapy for refractory orbital inflammation: Results of a phase 1/2, dose-ranging, randomized clinical trial. *JAMA Ophthalmol.* **2014**, *132*, 572–578. [CrossRef]
15. Kurz, P.A.; Suhler, E.B.; Choi, D.; Rosenbaum, J.T. Rituximab for treatment of ocular inflammatory disease: A series of four cases. *Br. J. Ophthalmol.* **2009**, *93*, 546–548. [CrossRef]
16. Abell, R.G.; Patrick, A.; Rooney, K.G.; McKelvie, P.A.; McNab, A.A. Complete resolution of idiopathic sclerosing orbital inflammation after treatment with rituximab. *Ocul. Immunol. Inflamm.* **2015**, *23*, 176–179. [CrossRef]
17. Wu, K.Y.; Kulbay, M.; Daigle, P.; Nguyen, B.H.; Tran, S.D. Nonspecific Orbital Inflammation (NSOI): Unraveling the Molecular Pathogenesis, Diagnostic Modalities, and Therapeutic Interventions. *Int. J. Mol. Sci.* **2024**, *25*, 1553. [CrossRef]
18. Yesiltas, Y.S.; Gunduz, A.K. Idiopathic Orbital Inflammation: Review of Literature and New Advances. *Middle East. Afr. J. Ophthalmol.* **2018**, *25*, 71–80. [CrossRef]
19. Arysait, O.; Tiraset, N.; Preechawai, P.; Kayasut, K.; Sanghan, N.; Sittivarakul, W. IgG4-related disease in patients with idiopathic orbital inflammation. *BMC Ophthalmol.* **2021**, *21*, 356. [CrossRef]

20. Kubota, T.; Katayama, M.; Nishimura, R.; Moritani, S. Long-term outcomes of ocular adnexal lesions in IgG4-related ophthalmic disease. *Br. J. Ophthalmol.* **2020**, *104*, 345–349. [CrossRef]
21. Detiger, S.E.; Karim, A.F.; Verdijk, R.M.; van Hagen, P.M.; van Laar, J.A.M.; Paridaens, D. The treatment outcomes in IgG4-related orbital disease: A systematic review of the literature. *Acta Ophthalmol.* **2019**, *97*, 451–459. [CrossRef]
22. Ng, C.C.; Sy, A.; Cunningham, E.T., Jr. Rituximab for treatment of non-infectious and non-malignant orbital inflammatory disease. *J. Ophthalmic Inflamm. Infect.* **2021**, *11*, 24. [CrossRef] [PubMed]
23. Abou-Hanna, J.J.; Tiu Teo, H.M.; Thangavel, R.; Elner, V.M.; Demirci, H. Long-term follow up of systemic rituximab therapy as first-line and salvage therapy for idiopathic orbital inflammation and review of the literature. *Orbit* **2022**, *41*, 297–304. [CrossRef]
24. Hatton, M.P.; Rubin, P.A.; Foster, C.S. Successful treatment of idiopathic orbital inflammation with mycophenolate mofetil. *Am. J. Ophthalmol.* **2005**, *140*, 916–918. [CrossRef]
25. Joshi, L.; Tanna, A.; McAdoo, S.P.; Medjeral-Thomas, N.; Taylor, S.R.; Sandhu, G.; Tarzi, R.M.; Pusey, C.D.; Lightman, S. Long-term Outcomes of Rituximab Therapy in Ocular Granulomatosis with Polyangiitis: Impact on Localized and Nonlocalized Disease. *Ophthalmology* **2015**, *122*, 1262–1268. [CrossRef]
26. Umehara, H.; Okazaki, K.; Kawa, S.; Takahashi, H.; Goto, H.; Matsui, S.; Ishizaka, N.; Akamizu, T.; Sato, Y.; Kawano, M.; et al. The 2020 revised comprehensive diagnostic (RCD) criteria for IgG4-RD. *Mod Rheumatol* **2021**, *31*, 529–533. [CrossRef]
27. Garrity, J.A.; Coleman, A.W.; Matteson, E.L.; Eggenberger, E.R.; Waitzman, D.M. Treatment of recalcitrant idiopathic orbital inflammation (chronic orbital myositis) with infliximab. *Am. J. Ophthalmol.* **2004**, *138*, 925–930. [CrossRef] [PubMed]
28. Yan, J.; Wu, P. Idiopathic orbital myositis. *J. Craniofac Surg.* **2014**, *25*, 884–887. [CrossRef]
29. Mombaerts, I.; Schlingemann, R.O.; Goldschmeding, R.; Koornneef, L. Are systemic corticosteroids useful in the management of orbital pseudotumors? *Ophthalmology* **1996**, *103*, 521–528. [CrossRef]
30. Carruth, B.P.; Wladis, E.J. Inflammatory modulators and biologic agents in the treatment of idiopathic orbital inflammation. *Curr. Opin. Ophthalmol.* **2012**, *23*, 420–426. [CrossRef]
31. Hougardy, D.M.; Peterson, G.M.; Bleasel, M.D.; Randall, C.T. Is enough attention being given to the adverse effects of corticosteroid therapy? *J. Clin. Pharm. Ther.* **2000**, *25*, 227–234. [CrossRef] [PubMed]
32. Bielory, L.; Frohman, L.P. Low-dose cyclosporine therapy of granulomatous optic neuropathy and orbitopathy. *Ophthalmology* **1991**, *98*, 1732–1736. [CrossRef] [PubMed]
33. Espinoza, G.M. Orbital inflammatory pseudotumors: Etiology, differential diagnosis, and management. *Curr. Rheumatol. Rep.* **2010**, *12*, 443–447. [CrossRef] [PubMed]
34. Eagle, K.; King, A.; Fisher, C.; Souhami, R. Cyclophosphamide induced remission in relapsed, progressive idiopathic orbital inflammation ('Pseudotumour'). *Clin. Oncol. (R. Coll. Radiol.)* **1995**, *7*, 402–404. [CrossRef]
35. Smith, J.R.; Rosenbaum, J.T. A role for methotrexate in the management of non-infectious orbital inflammatory disease. *Br. J. Ophthalmol.* **2001**, *85*, 1220–1224. [CrossRef] [PubMed]
36. Schafranski, M.D. Idiopathic orbital inflammatory disease successfully treated with rituximab. *Clin. Rheumatol.* **2009**, *28*, 225–226. [CrossRef]
37. Ashkenazy, N.; Saboo, U.S.; Abraham, A.; Ronconi, C.; Cao, J.H. Successful treatment with infliximab after adalimumab failure in pediatric noninfectious uveitis. *J. AAPOS* **2019**, *23*, 151.e1–151.e5. [CrossRef]
38. Mokhtech, M.; Nurkic, S.; Morris, C.G.; Mendenhall, N.P.; Mendenhall, W.M. Radiotherapy for Orbital Pseudotumor: The University of Florida Experience. *Cancer Investig.* **2018**, *36*, 330–337. [CrossRef]
39. Lee, J.H.; Kim, Y.S.; Yang, S.W.; Cho, W.K.; Lee, S.N.; Lee, K.J.; Ryu, M.R.; Jang, H.S. Radiotherapy with or without surgery for patients with idiopathic sclerosing orbital inflammation refractory or intolerant to steroid therapy. *Int. J. Radiat. Oncol. Biol. Phys.* **2012**, *84*, 52–58. [CrossRef]
40. Campochiaro, C.; Ramirez, G.A.; Bozzolo, E.P.; Lanzillotta, M.; Berti, A.; Baldissera, E.; Dagna, L.; Praderio, L.; Scotti, R.; Tresoldi, M.; et al. IgG4-related disease in Italy: Clinical features and outcomes of a large cohort of patients. *Scand. J. Rheumatol.* **2016**, *45*, 135–145. [CrossRef]
41. Khosroshahi, A.; Wallace, Z.S.; Crowe, J.L.; Akamizu, T.; Azumi, A.; Carruthers, M.N.; Chari, S.T.; Della-Torre, E.; Frulloni, L.; Goto, H.; et al. International Consensus Guidance Statement on the Management and Treatment of IgG4-Related Disease. *Arthritis Rheumatol.* **2015**, *67*, 1688–1699. [CrossRef]
42. Hart, P.A.; Topazian, M.D.; Witzig, T.E.; Clain, J.E.; Gleeson, F.C.; Klebig, R.R.; Levy, M.J.; Pearson, R.K.; Petersen, B.T.; Smyrk, T.C.; et al. Treatment of relapsing autoimmune pancreatitis with immunomodulators and rituximab: The Mayo Clinic experience. *Gut* **2013**, *62*, 1607–1615. [CrossRef]
43. Mannor, G.E.; Rose, G.E.; Moseley, I.F.; Wright, J.E. Outcome of orbital myositis: Clinical features associated with recurrence. *Ophthalmology* **1997**, *104*, 409–414. [CrossRef]
44. Halimi, E.; Rosenberg, R.; Wavreille, O.; Bouckehove, S.; Franquet, N.; Labalette, P. Présentation clinique et prise en charge des myosites aiguës dans les inflammations orbitaires non spécifiques [Clinical features and management of acute myositis in idiopathic orbital inflammation]. *J. Fr. Ophtalmol.* **2013**, *36*, 567–574 (in French). [CrossRef]
45. Montagnese, F.; Wenninger, S.; Schoser, B. Orbiting around the orbital myositis: Clinical features, differential diagnosis and therapy. *J. Neurol.* **2016**, *263*, 631–640. [CrossRef] [PubMed]
46. Kang, M.S.; Yang, H.K.; Kim, N.; Hwang, J.-M. Clinical Features of Ocular Motility in Idiopathic Orbital Myositis. *J. Clin. Med.* **2020**, *9*, 1165. [CrossRef]

47. Andrew, N.H.; Kearney, D.; Sladden, N.; McKelvie, P.; Wu, A.; Sun, M.T.; McNab, A.; Selva, D. Idiopathic Dacryoadenitis: Clinical Features, Histopathology, and Treatment Outcomes. *Am. Jounral Ophthalmol.* **2016**, *163*, 148–153.E1. [CrossRef]
48. Kubota, T.; Iwakoshi, A. Clinical heterogeneity between two subgroups of patients with idiopathic orbital inflammation. *BMJ Open Ophthalmol.* **2022**, *7*, e001005. [CrossRef]
49. Yuen, S.J.A.; Rubin, P.A.D. Idiopathic Orbital Inflammation: Distribution, Clinical Features, and Treatment Outcome. *Arch. Ophthalmol.* **2003**, *121*, 491–499. [CrossRef] [PubMed]

Disclaimer/Publisher's Note: The statements, opinions and data contained in all publications are solely those of the individual author(s) and contributor(s) and not of MDPI and/or the editor(s). MDPI and/or the editor(s) disclaim responsibility for any injury to people or property resulting from any ideas, methods, instructions or products referred to in the content.

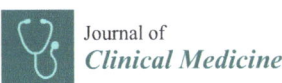

Article

Clinical Significance of the Inferomedial Orbital Strut in Orbital Blowout Fractures: Incidence of Symptomatic Diplopia in a Fractured vs. Intact Strut

Steffani Krista Someda, Hidetaka Miyazaki, Hirohiko Kakizaki and Yasuhiro Takahashi *

Department of Oculoplastic, Orbital & Lacrimal Surgery, Aichi Medical University Hospital, Nagakute 480-1195, Aichi, Japan; steffsomeda@gmail.com (S.K.S.); miyaosur@gmail.com (H.M.); cosme_geka@yahoo.co.jp (H.K.)
* Correspondence: yasuhiro_tak@yahoo.co.jp; Tel.: +81-561-62-3311 (ext. 12314)

Abstract: Background/Objectives: This study aims to compare the clinical findings, particularly symptomatic diplopia, associated with an inferomedial orbital strut fracture versus intact strut and to determine the clinical significance of the inferomedial orbital strut in patients with orbital floor and medial orbital wall fractures. **Methods**: A 10-year retrospective observational study involving orbital blowout fracture cases was conducted in our institution. Patients with fractures of the orbital floor medial to the infraorbital groove and medial orbital wall, as seen on computed tomography (CT) scans, were included in this study. Patients with concomitant orbital rim fracture and those with old orbital fractures were excluded. Fracture of the inferomedial orbital strut was diagnosed via coronal CT images and patients were classified into those with an inferomedial orbital strut fracture and those without. **Results**: A total of 231 orbits from 230 patients was included in the study (fractured strut on 78 sides and intact strut on 153 sides). Approximately 2/3 of patients in both groups had the field of binocular single vision in primary position upon first examination ($p = 0.717$). Patients with strut fractures demonstrated only comminuted or open fractures, while those without strut fractures showed diverse fracture patterns ($p < 0.001$). **Conclusions**: Inferomedial orbital strut fracture does not automatically result in diplopia in patients with orbital blowout fractures. The integrity of the orbital periosteum plays a more essential role in hampering extraocular muscle displacement, thereby preventing symptomatic diplopia in these patients.

Keywords: blowout fracture; diplopia; inferomedial orbital strut; medial orbital wall fracture; orbital floor fracture

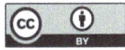

1. Introduction

In 1992, Goldberg et al. introduced the anatomical concept of the inferomedial orbital strut, which was utilized during transconjunctival orbital decompression in patients with dysthyroid optic neuropathy in order to prevent ocular dystopia [1]. This study was conducted based on the findings of Long and Baylis who documented patients having marked postoperative hypoglobus following inferomedial orbital decompression surgery [2]. In 1999, Burm et al. also documented the presence of a "bony buttress" demarcating the medial and inferior orbital walls, further implicating its importance in supporting these orbital walls and to prevent diplopia caused by globe displacement [3]. And in the year 2000, Kim et al. published a more comprehensive study on this inferomedial orbital bone structure [4]. This strut of bone, measuring 5 to 7 mm at its widest anterior portion, was found to be anchored firmly at the orbital rim and supported by the medial wall of the maxillary antrum [1,4]. Apart from their finding that ocular dystopia was prevented when the strut was utilized and left intact, this study concluded that the bony inferomedial structure can serve as a medial supporting "ledge" for orbital floor reconstruction [1,4], and this concept holds actual truth. Reconstruction of the medial and inferior orbital walls, in fact, uses the inferomedial strut as an important landmark in positioning the orbital implant of choice [5]. The fracture of this bony strut can, therefore, cause impending trouble for orbital wall reconstruction [5–7]. Furthermore, previous studies on orbital decompression have reported an increased incidence of postoperative diplopia, or non-resolution of pre-existing diplopia, in patients whose inferomedial orbital struts were surgically removed [1,8–10]. The question now is whether the risk of clinically significant diplopia also increases in orbital blowout fracture patients with concomitant strut fractures.

A spontaneous clinical improvement in patients conservatively treated for orbital blowout fractures has been documented in the literature [11,12]. However, the significance of the inferomedial orbital strut in preventing fracture-related symptomatic diplopia has yet to be established. This study, therefore, aims to determine if a fracture of the inferomedial orbital strut would result in clinically significant diplopia, based on binocular single-vision (BSV) testing, in patients with inferior and medial orbital wall fractures, as well as to determine the type of fractures associated with an inferomedial orbital strut fracture.

2. Materials and Methods

This was a retrospective, observational study including all patients with orbital fractures who were referred to our service from May 2013 to April 2023. Our hospital introduced an electronic medical chart system in May 2013. Patients with fractures of the orbital floor medial to the infraorbital groove and medial orbital wall were included in this study. Patients with a concomitant orbital rim fracture, i.e., impure orbital fracture, and those with old orbital fractures were excluded from this study.

The data on age, sex, affected side, the time of examination, causes of injury, concomitant ocular/periocular injuries, presence or absence of infraorbital nerve hypoesthesia, fields of BSV examined on the first visit, and surgery were collected. Causes of injury were classified as follows according to our previous study [13]: sports, assault, fall, traffic accident, works, and others. The results of the field of BSV were classified into 5 categories (B1 to B5), according to our previous study [13], as follows: B1, within normal range ($\pm 2 \times$ standard deviation); B2, the field of BSV reaches at least 20 degrees superiorly, 40 degrees inferiorly, and 30 degrees horizontally; B3, a smaller field of BSV than B2 but includes primary gaze; B4, the field of BSV does not include primary gaze; and B5, cannot obtain the field of BSV in any direction of gaze. Data on the presence of enophthalmos were not collected because orbital soft tissue edema caused by trauma prevents accurate Hertel exophthalmometric measurements. Data on postoperative findings were not collected due to several reasons: (1) not all patients included in the study underwent surgical reduction; (2) surgeries were performed by different surgeons; (3) there were different follow-up periods among the patients; and (4) some patients were lost to follow-up after the surgery.

Indications for the surgical repair of orbital fractures in our department were determined based on patient age, the field of BSV, and risk of enophthalmos. Surgical reduction was strongly recommended to patients presenting with a field of BSV at B3 or worse, as well as to patients with a large medial orbital wall fracture susceptible to enophthalmos. Surgery was also recommended to young patients, even with the grade of B2, due to their relatively wider range of activity, which required a wider field of BSV, whereas elderly patients had a narrower range of activity and a higher risk of iatrogenic ophthalmoplegia after surgery. Hence, conservative management was more advisable for elderly patients.

Axial and coronal CT images with bone and soft tissue window algorithms were obtained from all patients. Inferomedial strut fractures were diagnosed in cases with apparent strut fractures shown on coronal CT images (Figure 1a,b) or when the distance from the junction between the orbital floor and medial orbital wall and nasal septum was apparently shorter on the affected side (Figure 1c). Orbital fracture patterns, sites, entrapped orbital soft tissues in cases with trapdoor fractures, and concomitant nasal bone fractures were examined. Fracture patterns were classified into comminuted/open, hinged, trapdoor, and linear fractures [14]. The presence or absence of fractures of the orbital floor lateral to the infraorbital groove (Figure 1d) was checked [15]. Entrapped orbital soft tissues in cases with a trapdoor orbital fracture included the extraocular muscles and orbital fat.

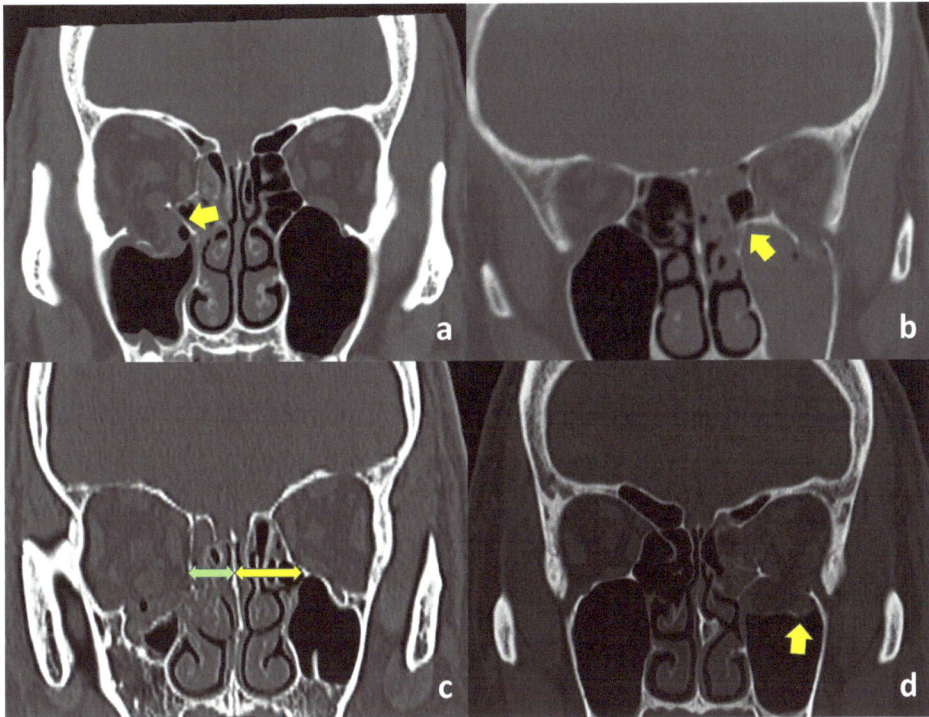

Figure 1. Computed tomographic (CT) findings. (**a**). The inferomedial orbital strut is not fractured (arrow). (**b**). The inferomedial orbital strut is fractured (arrow). (**c**). The distance from the junction between the orbital floor and medial orbital wall and nasal septum is shorter on the affected side (green arrow), compared to the unaffected side (yellow arrow). (**d**). The orbital floor lateral to the infraorbital groove (arrow) is fractured.

Patient age was expressed as means ± standard deviations. Patients were classified into those with and without inferomedial orbital strut fractures. Patient age was compared between the groups using the Student's t-test. A chi-squared test was employed to compare the categorical variables between the groups. All statistical analyses were performed using SPSS™ version 26 software (IBM Japan, Tokyo, Japan). Two-tailed p values < 0.05 were deemed to indicate statistical significance.

3. Results

Data on patient characteristics and clinical and radiological findings are shown in Tables 1–3. Among 1093 sides from 1074 patients with pure orbital fractures, 231 sides from 230 patients with fractures of the orbital floor medial to the infraorbital nerve and medial orbital wall (mean age: 40.8 ± 23.1 years; 160 males and 70 females) were included. All patients were Japanese. The inferomedial orbital strut was fractured on 78 sides in 78 patients, and the strut was intact on 153 sides in 153 patients. One patient with a bilateral orbital floor and medial orbital wall fractures showed an inferomedial orbital strut fracture on one side and no strut fracture on the other side.

Table 1. Data on patient characteristics.

Items	Total	Strut Fracture	No Strut Fracture	p Value
Number of patients/sides	230/231	78/78 (33.8%)	153/153 (66.2%)	
Age (years)	40.8 ± 23.1	43.3 ± 22.1	39.6 ± 23.5	0.240
M/F	160 (69.6%)/70 (30.4%)	56 (71.8%)/22 (28.2%)	105 (68.6%)/48 (31.4%)	0.653
R/L	109 (47.2%)/122 (52.8%)	35 (44.9%)/43 (55.1%)	74 (48.4%)/79 (51.6%)	0.677
Time of examination (days)	8.0 ± 5.3	7.7 ± 5.5	8.3 ± 5.0	0.499
Causes of injury				
Sports	69 (29.9%)	19 (24.4%)	50 (32.7%)	
Assault	34 (14.7%)	12 (15.4%)	22 (14.4%)	
Fall	81 (35.1%)	31 (39.7%)	50 (32.7%)	0.638
Traffic accident	25 (10.8%)	10 (12.8%)	15 (9.8%)	
Work	8 (3.5%)	3 (3.8%)	5 (3.3%)	
Others	14 (6.1%)	3 (3.8%)	11 (7.2%)	

M, male; F, female; R, right; L, left.

Table 2. Data on clinical findings.

Items	Total	Strut Fracture	No Strut Fracture	p Value
Number of patients with concomitant ocular/periocular injuries (some overlapped)	45 (19.6%)	21 (26.9%)	24 (15.7%)	0.053
Hyphema	8	5	3	
Iritis	1	0	1	
Vitreous hemorrhage	2	1	1	
Retinal hemorrhage	1	1	0	
Serous macular detachment	2	0	2	
Maculopathy	1	1	0	
Commotio retinae	13	5	8	
Retinal tear	1	1	0	
Macular hole	3	2	1	
Choroidal rupture	1	1	0	
Globe rupture	3	0	3	
Orbital compartment syndrome	1	0	1	
Traumatic mydriasis	3	1	2	
Eyelid laceration	4	3	1	
Traumatic ptosis	8	5	3	
Floppy eyelid	1	1	0	
Canalicular laceration	1	0	1	
Nasolacrimal canal fracture	2	1	1	
Traumatic superior oblique palsy	1	0	1	
Optic nerve canal fracture	1	1	0	
Infraorbital nerve hypoesthesia	69 (29.9%)	26 (33.3%)	43 (28.1%)	0.449
Field of BSV				
B1	32 (15.2%)	8 (11.3%)	24 (17.1%)	
B2	57 (27.0%)	18 (25.4%)	39 (27.9%)	
B3	68 (32.2%)	24 (33.8%)	44 (31.4%)	0.717
B4	25 (11.8%)	9 (12.7%)	16 (11.4%)	
B5	29 (13.7%)	12 (16.9%)	17 (12.1%)	
Unmeasurable	19 *	7	13	
Number of patients who underwent surgery	144 (62.6%)	55 (70.5%)	89 (58.2%)	0.085

BSV, binocular single vision. * One case had a strut fracture on one side and no strut fracture on the other side.

Patient age, male-and-female ratio, right-and-left ratio, the time of examination, and ratio of causes of injury were not significantly different between the groups ($p > 0.050$). Concomitant ocular/periocular injuries tended to more frequently occur in patients with strut fractures (26.9% vs. 15.7%; $p = 0.053$). The incidence of infraorbital nerve hypoesthesia was not different between the groups ($p = 0.449$).

Table 3. Data on radiological findings.

Items	Total	Strut Fracture	No Strut Fracture	p Value
Fracture patterns (floor/medial)				
Comminuted/comminuted	129 (55.8%)	78 (100.0%)	51 (33.3%)	
Hinged/hinged	30 (13.0%)	0	30 (19.6%)	
Trapdoor/trapdoor	18 (7.8%)	0	18 (11.8%)	
Linear/linear	2 (0.9%)	0	2 (1.3%)	
Comminuted/hinged	12 (5.2%)	0	12 (7.8%)	
Comminuted/trapdoor	13 (5.6%)	0	13 (8.5%)	
Comminuted/linear	1 (0.4%)	0	1 (0.7%)	<0.001
Hinged/comminuted	5 (2.2%)	0	5 (3.3%)	
Hinged/trapdoor	6 (2.6%)	0	6 (3.9%)	
Hinged/linear	1 (0.4%)	0	1 (0.7%)	
Trapdoor/comminuted	3 (1.3%)	0	3 (2.0%)	
Trapdoor/hinged	4 (1.7%)	0	4 (2.6%)	
Linear/comminuted	4 (1.7%)	0	4 (2.6%)	
Linear/trapdoor	3 (1.3%)	0	3 (2.0%)	
Concomitant orbital floor fracture lateral to infraorbital groove	36 (16.9%)	15 (19.2%)	21 (13.7%)	0.338
Incarcerated tissues				
Inferior rectus muscle	1 (0.4%)	0	1 (0.7%)	
Inferior rectus muscle (floor) + orbital fat (medial)	1 (0.4%)	0	1 (0.7%)	<0.001
Orbital fat (floor and/or medial)	45 (19.5%)	0	45 (29.4%)	
Number of patients with concomitant nasal bone fracture	12 (5.2%)	8 (10.3%)	4 (2.6%)	0.024

Approximately 2/3 patients in both groups had the field of BSV in the primary position ($\geq$B3) on the first examination ($p = 0.717$). A total of 19 patients with "unmeasurable" BSV resulted from either having their vision totally obscured due to the ocular injury or a lack of comprehension in pediatric patients of BSV testing. However, a larger number of patients with strut fractures tended to undergo surgical reductions in orbital fractures, compared to those without strut fractures (70.5% vs. 58.2%; $p = 0.085$).

With regard to the radiological findings, although fracture patterns had variety in patients without strut fractures, patients with strut fractures demonstrated only comminuted/open fractures ($p < 0.001$). According to this finding, all 46 patients with orbital trapdoor fractures did not sustain strut fractures ($p < 0.001$). Although the incidence of concomitant orbital floor fractures lateral to the infraorbital groove was slightly higher in patients with strut fractures (19.2% vs. 13.7%), the difference did not show statistical significance ($p = 0.338$). Concomitant nasal bone fractures were more frequently shown in patients with strut fractures (10.3% vs. 2.6%; $p = 0.024$).

4. Discussion

Symptomatic diplopia associated with orbital blowout fractures was first documented in 1957 by Converse and Smith [16]. This usually occurs due to ocular deviation caused by the entrapment of one or more extraocular muscles [16]. The fracture can also lead to the direct injury of the muscle, i.e., laceration, disinsertion, intramuscular hemorrhage, or damage to the nerve controlling eye movement [17]. In fractures involving more than half of the orbital floor, there is also the possibility of the hypoglobus likewise resulting to diplopia [2,16]. Retrospective studies published within the past decade have reported on the incidence of diplopia caused by orbital blowout fractures to be ranging from 20% to as high as 83% [11,12,18]. However, these studies did not indicate the presence of strut fractures. In our previous studies, the incidence of inferomedial strut fractures in patients with orbital blowout fractures was found to be 9% of the sample population (45 out of 475 cases) in one study and 6% (41 out of 671 orbits) in another study [13,19]. Although the incidence rates appear to have insignificant numbers, the implications of these types of fractures will nonetheless aid the clinician in managing such cases.

In our present study, 21 patients with strut fractures (26.9%) were found to have BSV worse than B3, which indicates the presence of diplopia on the primary position of gaze, while 33 patients presenting with similar BSV outcomes had intact inferomedial struts (21.6%). Although the group with fractured struts had a slightly higher frequency of diplopia on primary gaze, statistical analysis showed no significant difference between the fractured strut group and the intact strut group. According to previous studies on medial orbital wall decompression, diplopia occurred when the inferomedial orbital strut was not utilized [4,14]. In contrast, our study has found that strut fractures do not necessarily result in diplopia in orbital blowout fractures. A study by Mansour et al. has similarly found that the involvement of the inferomedial strut is not predictive of the development of diplopia requiring surgical intervention for orbital blowout fractures [20]. Despite having intra-orbital contents herniating through the fracture site, the integrity of the periosteum may actually be more important in preventing clinically significant diplopia [14]. In patients with strut fractures but an intact periosteum, the periosteal layer seems to serve as a hammock that keeps the orbital contents, especially the extraocular muscles, from becoming displaced or incarcerated. This is important for maintaining adequate ocular movement and preventing diplopia, which is mainly caused by the entrapment of extraocular muscles and the intrinsic fibrosis of adjacent fibrofatty tissue secondary to trauma [21].

The presumptive diagnosis of periosteal tear can be made via CT or MRI when the herniated orbital contents do not show a smooth margin [6] or when prolapsed orbital fat crosses over the area of bone fragmentation [21]. However, the presence of a periosteal tear can be quite difficult to ascertain based simply on the radiologic configuration of orbital fat herniation. As such, surgical exploration is still necessary to provide a definitive diagnosis and to address the cause of the diplopia. Although the question of whether muscle impingement can still occur, despite having an intact periosteum, is yet to be investigated, the integrity of the periosteum is definitely much more important than the integrity of the inferomedial orbital strut in the prevention of clinically significant diplopia.

In the fractured strut group, the percentage of patients who underwent surgery was also noted to be higher (70.5%) as compared to the intact strut group (58.2%). Damage to the inferomedial strut could have led to an inadvertent expansion of the orbital space, resulting in clinically significant enophthalmos necessitating surgical intervention [22–24]. On the other hand, some of the patients in the intact strut group presented with only fat incarceration and no significant enophthalmos. For this reason, surgery was not indicated.

In the coronal view of orbital imaging, the inferomedial orbital strut can be identified as the bony junction between the medial and inferior orbital walls (Figure 1) [25]. The most common site of fracture, based on our previous study, was found to be the orbital floor medial to the infraorbital nerve [13]. This inferomedial portion of the bony orbit appears to be thinner than the portion of the orbital floor lateral to the infraorbital nerve [14], where the maxillary and zygomatic bones meet, and the integrity of the inferomedial strut becomes even more important to maintain support of the orbital contents. As a buttress of the orbit, the fracture of the inferomedial orbital strut, hence, can be confirmed on imaging when there is a shortening of the distance between this bony junction and the nasal septum (Figure 1c).

Kim et al., in their anatomic study of the inferomedial orbital strut and its clinical implications in globe dystopia after orbital decompression surgery, found that some patients may be prone to concomitant strut fractures due to the presence of pneumatization by the maxillary sinus anteriorly and ethmoid sinus posteriorly [4]. Based on a study by de Silva and Rose, strut fractures were also more common in African (37%) and Asian (30%) patients as compared to the Caucasian patients (13%), probably due to either a greater impact from the trauma or weaker strut associated with these races [26]. Although a recent study by Chan et al. found no significant inter-ethnic variations in the medial orbital wall among Caucasians, the study, nonetheless, found that Chinese, Malays, and Indians had their posterior ethmoidal wall anterior to the posterior maxillary wall, as opposed to Caucasians who had their posterior maxillary wall anterior to the posterior ethmoidal wall [27]. Demographic factors, therefore, contribute to the higher incidence of inferomedial orbital strut fractures resulting from anatomical variations found in certain populations.

The results of the study show that the percentage of patients with ocular injuries is higher in the fractured orbital strut group (26.9%) as compared to the intact-strut group (15.7%). This result is consistent with our previous study showing a high prevalence of inferomedial orbital strut fractures in patients with both pure orbital fractures and lacrimal drainage system injuries [28]. The risk of ocular injuries is lower in patients with orbital blowout fractures, compared to those without fractures, because pressure on the globe at the moment of impact with a material escapes through the fracture site [14,29]. The finding of the present study may likely be due to a high-velocity or a greater force of impact causing both ocular injuries and the strut fractures in these group of patients.

With regards to the concomitant nasal bone fractures found more frequently in patients with strut fractures, this correlation can be explained by the buckling force of impact on the medial orbital rim [3], inevitably causing nasal bone fracture and possibly affecting the most fragile medial portion of the orbital strut.

This study found intact inferomedial orbital struts in 46 patients with orbital trapdoor fractures, although all patients in the fractured strut group showed comminuted or open fractures. A similar finding was reported in the 1999 study by Burm et al. [3]. The likelihood that trapdoor fractures tend to occur in younger patients can explain this phenomenon [14]. Higher bone elasticity found in younger patients decreases the risk of acquiring comminuted fractures [14,30,31], thereby decreasing the risk of concomitant damage to the orbital strut. Despite having all patients with trapdoor fractures in the intact strut group, there was no significant statistical difference in the frequency of symptomatic diplopia between the two study groups. This may be due to the inclusion of only two cases with inferior rectus muscle incarcerations in the intact strut group. Some patients presenting with only orbital fat incarceration do not experience diplopia [32,33]. The main cause of diplopia in cases with orbital fat incarceration is the concomitant incarceration of the inferior oblique muscle branch of the oculomotor nerve, and the incidence of this complication is found to be only 18% [14]. This low incidence may also explain why there is no significant difference in the frequency of symptomatic diplopia between the study groups.

This study has its limitations. For one, the study was performed in a single institution and included consecutive patients diagnosed with orbital blowout fractures. Therefore, randomization of the sample population was not achieved. Furthermore, all patients included were of Japanese descent. Although patient age and sex had no statistically significant difference among the study population, other demographic factors, such as race, can imply possible anatomical differences that may affect the generalizability of the study outcome [27,34]. Lastly, the study was retrospective in nature. The recommendation for future studies would be to conduct a prospective multi-center study that can also factor in populations with different ethnicities. In addition to this, the authors recommend further investigation of the likelihood of diplopia caused by orbital tissue incarceration in the absence of periosteal injury in orbital blowout fracture patients.

5. Conclusions

In conclusion, we compared clinical characteristics between patients with and without inferomedial orbital strut fractures. Although fracture patterns and frequency of ocular and periocular injuries tended to be different between the groups, fracture of the inferomedial orbital strut did not affect BSV findings in patients with orbital blowout fractures.

Author Contributions: Conceptualization, Y.T.; methodology, Y.T.; validation, Y.T.; formal analysis, S.K.S., H.M. and Y.T.; investigation, Y.T.; writing—original draft preparation, S.K.S.; writing—review and editing, H.M., H.K. and Y.T.; supervision, Y.T.; project administration, Y.T. All authors have read and agreed to the published version of the manuscript.

Funding: This research received no external funding.

Institutional Review Board Statement: The institutional review board (IRB) of Aichi Medical University Hospital approved this retrospective, observational study, which was conducted in accordance with the tenets of the Declaration of Helsinki and its later amendments (approval number, 2023-131).

Informed Consent Statement: The IRB granted a waiver of informed consent for this study based on the ethical guidelines for medical and health research involving human subjects established by the Japanese Ministry of Education, Culture, Sports, Science, and Technology; and by the Ministry of Health, Labour, and Welfare. The waiver was granted because the study was a retrospective chart review, not an interventional study. Nevertheless, at the request of the IRB, we published an outline of the study on the Aichi Medical University website that was available for public viewing, which also provided the patients an option to refuse to participate in the study, although none did. Personal identifiers were removed from the records prior to data analysis.

Data Availability Statement: Data supporting the results of this study are available upon request.

Conflicts of Interest: The authors declare no conflicts of interest.

References

1. Goldberg, R.A.; Shorr, N.; Cohen, M. The medial orbital strut in the prevention of postdecompression dystopia in dysthyroid ophthalmopathy. *Ophthalmic Plast. Reconstr. Surg.* **1992**, *8*, 32–34. [CrossRef]
2. Long, J.A.; Baylis, H.I. Hypoglobus following orbital decompression for dysthyroid ophthalmopathy. *Ophthalmic Plast. Recostr Surg.* **1990**, *6*, 185–189. [CrossRef]
3. Burm, J.S.; Chung, C.H.; Oh, S.J. Pure orbital blowout fracture: New concepts and importance of medial orbital blowout fracture. *Plast. Reconstr. Surg.* **1999**, *103*, 1839–1849. [CrossRef] [PubMed]
4. Kim, J.W.; Goldberg, R.A.; Shorr, N. The inferomedial orbital strut: An anatomic and radiographic study. *Ophthalmic Plast. Reconstr. Surg.* **2002**, *18*, 355–364. [CrossRef] [PubMed]
5. Hur, S.W.; Kim, S.E.; Chung, K.J.; Lee, J.H.; Kim, T.G.; Kim, Y.H. Combined orbital fractures: Surgical strategy of sequential repair. *Arch. Plast. Surg.* **2015**, *42*, 424–430. [CrossRef]
6. Kim, J.H.; Lee, I.G.; Lee, J.S.; Oh, D.Y.; Jun, Y.J.; Rhie, J.W.; Shim, J.H.; Moon, S.H. Restoration of the inferomedial orbital strut using a standardized three-dimensional printing implant. *J. Anat.* **2020**, *236*, 923–930. [CrossRef]
7. Park, T.H. The usefulness of the navigation system to reconstruct orbital wall fractures involving inferomedial orbital strut. *J. Clin. Med.* **2023**, *12*, 4968. [CrossRef]
8. Wright, E.D.; Davidson, J.; Codere, F.; Desrosiers, M. Endoscopic orbital decompression with preservation of an inferomedial bony strut: Minimization of postoperative diplopia. *J. Otolaryngol.* **1999**, *28*, 252–256.
9. Finn, A.P.; Bleier, B.; Cestari, D.M.; Kazlas, M.A.; Dagi, L.R.; Lefebvre, D.R.; Yoon, M.K.; Freitag, S.K. A retrospective review of orbital decompression for thyroid orbitopathy with endoscopic preservation of the inferomedial orbital bone strut. *Ophthalmic Plast. Reconstr. Surg.* **2017**, *33*, 334–339. [CrossRef]
10. Yao, W.C.; Sedaghat, A.R.; Yadav, P.; Fay, A.; Metson, R. Orbital decompression in the endoscopic age: The modified inferomedial orbital strut. *Otolaryngol. Head. Neck Surg.* **2016**, *154*, 963–969. [CrossRef]
11. Young, S.M.; Kim, Y.D.; Kim, S.W.; Jo, H.B.; Lang, S.S.; Cho, K.; Woo, K.I. Conservatively treated orbital blowout fractures: Spontaneous radiologic improvement. *Ophthalmology* **2018**, *125*, 938–944. [CrossRef] [PubMed]
12. Lin, C.H.; Lee, S.S.; Lin, I.W.; Su, W.J. Is surgery needed for diplopia after blowout fractures? A clarified algorithm to assist decision-making. *Plast. Reconstr. Surg. Glob. Open* **2022**, *10*, e4308. [CrossRef] [PubMed]
13. Takahashi, Y.; Nakakura, S.; Sabundayo, M.S.; Kitaguchi, Y.; Miyazaki, H.; Mito, H.; Kakizaki, H. Differences in common orbital blowout fracture sites by age. *Plast. Reconstr. Surg.* **2018**, *141*, 893e–901e. [CrossRef] [PubMed]
14. Valencia, M.R.P.; Miyazaki, H.; Ito, M.; Nishimura, K.; Kakizaki, H.; Takahashi, Y. Radiological findings of orbital blowout fractures: A review. *Orbit* **2021**, *40*, 98–109. [CrossRef] [PubMed]
15. Takahashi, Y.; Vaidya, A.; Kono, S.; Miyazaki, H.; Yokoyama, T.; Kakizaki, H. The relationship between orbital fracture patterns around the infraorbital groove and development of infraorbital hypoesthesia: A computed tomographic study. *Graefes Arch. Clin. Exp. Ophthalmol.* **2023**, *261*, 841–848. [CrossRef] [PubMed]
16. Converse, J.M.; Smith, B. Enophthalmos and diplopia in fractures of the orbital floor. *Br. J. Plast. Surg.* **1957**, *9*, 265–274. [CrossRef]
17. Braaksma-Besselink, Y.; Jellema, H.M. Orthoptic evaluation and treatment in orbital fractures. *Atlas Oral. Maxillofac. Surg. Clin. N. Am.* **2021**, *29*, 41–50. [CrossRef]
18. Bartoli, D.; Fadda, M.T.; Battisti, A.; Cassoni, A.; Pagnoni, M.; Riccardi, E.; Sanzi, M.; Valentini, V. Retrospective analysis of 301 patients with orbital floor fracture. *J. Craniomaxillofac Surg.* **2015**, *43*, 244–247. [CrossRef] [PubMed]
19. Sun, M.T.; Wu, W.; Watanabe, A.; Kakizaki, H.; Chen, B.; Ueda, K.; Katori, N.; Takahashi, Y.; Selva, D. Orbital blowout fracture location in Japanese and Chinese patients. *Jpn. J. Ophthalmol.* **2015**, *59*, 65–69. [CrossRef]
20. Mansour, T.N.; Rudolph, M.; Brown, D.; Mansour, N.; Taheri, M.R. Orbital blowout fractures: A novel CT measurement that can predict the likelihood of surgical management. *Am. J. Emerg. Med.* **2017**, *35*, 112–116. [CrossRef]

21. Harris, G.J.; Garcia, G.H.; Logani, S.C.; Murphy, M.L. Correlation of preoperative computed tomography and postoperative ocular motility in orbital blowout fractures. *Ophthalmic Plast. Reconstr. Surg.* **2000**, *16*, 179–187. [CrossRef]
22. Jeong, S.H.; Moon, K.C.; Namgoong, S.; Dhong, E.S.; Han, S.K. Anatomical reconstruction of extensive inferomedial blow-out fractures involving the inferomedial orbital strut using a single fan-shaped titanium-reinforced porous polyethylene plate. *J. Craniofac Surg.* **2023**, *34*, 1329–1334. [CrossRef]
23. Zhuang, A.; Wang, S.; Yuan, Q.; Li, Y.; Bi, X.; Shi, W. Surgical repair of large orbital floor and medial wall fractures with destruction of the inferomedial strut: Initial experience with a combined endoscopy navigation technique. *J. Plast. Reconstr. Aesthet. Surg.* **2023**, *77*, 104–110. [CrossRef] [PubMed]
24. Zhou, G.; Tu, Y.; Yu, B.; Wu, W. Endoscopic repair of combined orbital floor and medial wall fractures involving the inferomedial strut. *Eye* **2021**, *35*, 2763–2770. [CrossRef] [PubMed]
25. Tan, N.Y.Q.; Leong, Y.Y.; Lang, S.S.; Htoon, Z.M.; Young, S.M.; Sundar, G. Radiologic parameters of orbital bone remodeling in thyroid eye disease. *Investig. Ophthalmol. Vis. Sci.* **2017**, *58*, 2527–2533. [CrossRef]
26. De Silva, D.J.; Rose, G.E. Orbital blowout fractures and race. *Ophthalmology* **2011**, *118*, 1677–1680. [CrossRef] [PubMed]
27. Chan, M.A.; Ibrahim, F.; Kumaran, A.; Yong, K.; Chan, A.S.Y.; Shen, S. Ethnic variation in medial orbital wall anatomy and its implications for decompression surgery. *BMC Ophthalmol.* **2021**, *21*, 290. [CrossRef] [PubMed]
28. Someda, S.K.; Ambat, J.M.; Miyazaki, H.; Takahashi, Y. Incidence of pure orbital fractures with concomitant lacrimal drainage system injuries in the Japanese population: A retrospective study. *Semin. Ophthalmol.* **2024**; *online ahead of print*.
29. Zhou, B.; Uppuluri, A.; Zarbin, M.A.; Bhagat, N. Work-related ocular trauma in the United States: A National Trauma Databank study. *Graefes Arch. Clin. Exp. Ophthalmol.* **2023**, *261*, 2081–2088. [CrossRef] [PubMed]
30. Bhate, M.; Adewara, B.; Bothra, N. Strabismus in pediatric orbital wall fractures. *Indian. J. Ophthalmol.* **2023**, *71*, 973–976. [CrossRef]
31. Hsieh, P.J.; Liao, H.T. Outcome analysis of surgical timing in pediatric orbital trapdoor fracture with different entrapment contents: A retrospective study. *Children* **2022**, *9*, 398. [CrossRef]
32. Basnet, A.; Chug, A.; Simre, S.; Vyas, A.; Shrestha, S. Comprehensive management of pediatric orbital fractures: A case series and review of literature. *Cureus* **2024**, *16*, e57915. [CrossRef] [PubMed]
33. Su, Y.; Shen, Q.; Bi, X.; Lin, M.; Fan, X. Delayed surgical treatment of orbital trapdoor fracture in paediatric patients. *Br. J. Ophthalmol.* **2019**, *103*, 523–526. [CrossRef] [PubMed]
34. Moon, S.J.; Lee, W.J.; Roh, T.S.; Baek, W. Sex-related and racial variations in orbital floor anatomy. *Arch. Craniofac Surg.* **2020**, *21*, 219–224. [CrossRef] [PubMed]

Disclaimer/Publisher's Note: The statements, opinions and data contained in all publications are solely those of the individual author(s) and contributor(s) and not of MDPI and/or the editor(s). MDPI and/or the editor(s) disclaim responsibility for any injury to people or property resulting from any ideas, methods, instructions or products referred to in the content.

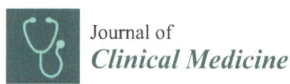 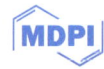

Article

Effects of Topical Anti-Glaucoma Medications on Outcomes of Endoscopic Dacryocystorhinostomy: Comparison with Age- and Sex-Matched Controls

Seong Eun Lee [1,2], Hyung Bin Lim [2,3], Seungjun Oh [2], Kibum Lee [1] and Sung Bok Lee [2,*]

1. Department of Ophthalmology, Chungbuk National University Hospital, College of Medicine, Chungbuk National University, Cheongju 28644, Republic of Korea; selee@cbnuh.or.kr (S.E.L.); kibum420@cbnuh.or.kr (K.L.)
2. Department of Ophthalmology, College of Medicine, Chungbuk National University, Daejeon 35015, Republic of Korea; 20210141@cnuh.co.kr (S.O.)
3. 1.0 Eye Clinic, Daejeon 34946, Republic of Korea; cromfans@hanmail.net (H.B.L.)
* Correspondence: sblee@cnu.ac.kr; Tel.: +82-4-2280-7604; Fax: +82-4-2255-3745

Abstract: Background: This study analyzed the effects of topical anti-glaucoma medications on the surgical outcomes of endoscopic dacryocystorhinostomy (EDCR) in nasolacrimal duct obstruction (NLDO). Methods: This retrospective study included patients who underwent EDCR for NLDO between September 2012 and April 2021. Thirty patients with topical anti-glaucoma medications and 90 age- and sex-matched controls were included. Results: The success rate of EDCR was higher in the control group than in the anti-glaucoma group (97.8% vs. 86.7%, $p = 0.034$). Univariate and multivariate logistic regression analyses identified prostaglandin analogs as the most influential risk factor for EDCR success among anti-glaucoma medication ingredients ($p = 0.005$). The success rate of the group containing all four anti-glaucoma medication ingredients was statistically significant ($p = 0.010$). The success rate was significantly different in the group of patients who used anti-glaucoma medication for >24 months ($p = 0.019$). When multiplying the number of drug ingredients by the duration in months, the group > 69 showed a significantly decreased success rate ($p = 0.022$). Multivariate logistic regression analysis identified the number of anti-glaucoma medications as the most significant risk factor for EDCR success (odds ratio, 0.437; 95% confidence interval, 0.247 to 0.772; $p = 0.004$). Conclusions: The authors suggest that the anti-glaucoma medications might cause NLDO and increase the failure rate after EDCR. Therefore, when performing EDCR in patients using topical anti-glaucoma medications, surgeons should consider the possibility of increased recurrence after EDCR in clinical outcomes.

Keywords: topical anti-glaucoma medication; endoscopic dacryocystorhinostomy; nasolacrimal duct obstruction; surgical outcome

Citation: Lee, S.E.; Lim, H.B.; Oh, S.; Lee, K.; Lee, S.B. Effects of Topical Anti-Glaucoma Medications on Outcomes of Endoscopic Dacryocystorhinostomy: Comparison with Age- and Sex-Matched Controls. *J. Clin. Med.* **2024**, *13*, 634. https://doi.org/10.3390/jcm13020634

Academic Editors: Kelvin Kam-Lung Chong and Renbing Jia

Received: 7 December 2023
Revised: 15 January 2024
Accepted: 19 January 2024
Published: 22 January 2024

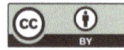

Copyright: © 2024 by the authors. Licensee MDPI, Basel, Switzerland. This article is an open access article distributed under the terms and conditions of the Creative Commons Attribution (CC BY) license (https://creativecommons.org/licenses/by/4.0/).

1. Introduction

The etiology of nasolacrimal duct obstruction (NLDO) has not been completely elucidated; however, idiopathic inflammation and fibrosis are known to lead to nasolacrimal duct (NLD) stenosis [1]. According to previous studies, 5–23% [2–4] of patients are pre-diagnosed with glaucoma when they are diagnosed with lacrimal drainage system obstruction. Anti-glaucoma medications may induce ocular surface diseases (OSD) such as conjunctival inflammation and subconjunctival fibrosis in patients [5,6]. The prevalence of OSD in patients with glaucoma due to the use of anti-glaucoma medications has been reported to be 17–52.3% in Asian populations and 40–60% in Western populations [5,7]. Active ingredients, preservatives, and excipients of anti-glaucoma medications are thought to cause ocular surface toxicity [3,7,8]. Several studies have inferred that anti-glaucoma medications may induce inflammation and fibrosis in the NLD mucosa, like how they affect the ocular surface, potentially leading to NLDO development [3,9].

Topical anti-glaucoma medications may also have a similar mechanism, affecting the newly created drainage pathway after dacryocystorhinostomy (DCR) and potentially influencing surgical outcomes. Therefore, when performing DCR on patients with concomitant glaucoma who have been using anti-glaucoma medications, it is important to consider the potential impact on surgical outcomes. Di Maria et al. [9] inferred that anti-glaucoma medications may damage the spiral fibers of the mucous membrane of the lacrimal system, induce fibrosis via a pro-inflammatory mechanism, and subsequently lead to decreased propulsive ability after DCR. This study aimed to compare the surgical success rates of patients using anti-glaucoma medications with those of an age- and sex-matched control group to investigate the impact of anti-glaucoma medications on DCR.

2. Materials and Methods

A retrospective review of the medical records of 795 patients who underwent endoscopic dacryocystorhinostomy (EDCR) procedures for NLDO at Chungnam National University Hospital between September 2012 and April 2021 was conducted. Patients who did not exhibit severe alterations in the osteomeatal complex, which could potentially affect the success rate of EDCR, were enrolled based on orbital computed tomography (CT) scans to standardize the surgical procedure. Severe scar formation or synechia resulting from trauma, tumors, or previous operations, potentially contributing to the failure of DCR, were excluded. During this period, 30 patients (3.8%) had a history of receiving topical anti-glaucoma medications. We included an age- and sex-matched control group of 90 patients.

Patients with glaucoma underwent additional ophthalmic examinations, including Goldmann applanation tonometry, fundus photography (TRC-NW8 fundus camera; Topcon Medical Systems, Tokyo, Japan), SD-OCT (Cirrus HD OCT; Carl Zeiss Meditec, Dublin, CA, USA), and the 24-2 Swedish Interactive Threshold Algorithm standard automated visual field test (Humphrey Visual Field Analyzer; Carl Zeiss Meditec, Dublin, CA, USA). Glaucoma was diagnosed based on glaucomatous optic disc changes and a reproducible glaucomatous visual field (VF) defect on Humphrey perimetry. Glaucomatous optic disc changes were defined as follows: diffuse or focal rim thinning, cupping, or retinal nerve fiber layer defects with corresponding VF defects. Glaucomatous VF defects were defined if they met two of the following three criteria: the presence of a cluster of three points on a pattern deviation probability plot at $p < 0.05$, one of which was at $p < 0.01$, a pattern standard deviation at $p < 0.05$, or glaucoma hemifield test results outside normal limits [10–12].

Anatomical success was defined as the observation of water passage during lacrimal irrigation with an open ostium confirmed through nasal endoscopy. The minimum required follow-up period was 6 months after surgery. The exclusion criteria were as follows: uncertain anti-glaucoma medication history; change in anti-glaucoma medications 6 months before EDCR surgery; less than 6 months of follow-up after EDCR surgery; patients who developed increased intraocular pressure as steroid responders after EDCR; history of congenital obstruction; eyelid margin malposition; previous lacrimal drainage system surgery; ocular or periocular trauma; history of systemic chemotherapy; and orbital radiotherapy. The study protocol was approved by the Institutional Review Board of the Chungnam National University Hospital (IRB no. 2023-03-016) and adhered to the tenets of the Declaration of Helsinki.

2.1. Surgical Technique

All surgeries were performed under general anesthesia by a single experienced surgeon. A gauze soaked in 1:10,000 epinephrine was packed into the middle meatus to decongest the nasal mucosa. After upper punctum dilatation, a 23-gauge vitrectomy light pipe was inserted through the upper canaliculus into the lacrimal sac. Lidocaine with 1:100,000 epinephrine was injected into the nasal mucosa at the lacrimal fossa, where the lacrimal sac was located. The nasal mucosa was incised using an elevator and removed using ethmoid forceps. A Kerrison rongeur was used to remove the bone and expose the lacrimal sac. The lacrimal sac was tented using a light pipe and excised using a crescent blade. After removing the lacrimal sac using ethmoid forceps, lacrimal irrigation was performed to confirm the patency of the lacrimal passage. Bicanalicular silicone tube intubation was performed, and the anastomosis site was packed with biodegradable synthetic polyurethane foam Nasopore (Polyganics, Groningen, The Netherlands).

Postoperatively, all patients were prescribed eye drops (topical antibiotics and steroids) and budesonide nasal spray. Follow-up examinations were performed at 1 and 2 weeks and at 1, 2, 3, 4, and 6 months after surgery. The silicone tube was removed three months after surgery, and lacrimal irrigation was performed at each visit.

2.2. Main Outcome Measures

The types, durations, and total ingredient numbers of topical anti-glaucoma medications, along with the EDCR surgical outcomes, were reviewed in detail. If the topical anti-glaucoma medication ingredients were changed, the analysis was based on the ingredients used during the 6-month period immediately before surgery. To compare the effects of drug ingredients, we counted the ingredients included in the fixed-combination anti-glaucoma medications separately. When two ingredients, brimonidine and timolol, were mixed in one bottle, the number of drugs was counted as two. To quantify the impact of the long-term use of a single ingredient versus the short-term use of multiple drug ingredients, we multiplied the number of eye drop ingredients by the duration in months.

2.3. Statistical Analysis

Statistical analyses were performed using SPSS statistical software (version 23.0; IBM Corp., Armonk, NY, USA) and the R statistical package (version 3.5.0; R Foundation for Statistical Computing, Vienna, Austria). The independent t-test, chi-square test, and Fisher's exact test were used to analyze baseline demographics. Univariate and multivariate logistic regression analyses were performed to evaluate the relationship between the ingredients of anti-glaucoma medications and the EDCR success rate and the risk factors associated with the EDCR success rate. Because of multicollinearity problem, stepwise backward elimination was performed to identify the independent factors. Fisher's exact test was used to compare the EDCR success rate according to the number of ingredients, duration of glaucoma treatment, and the product of the number of ingredients multiplied by duration in months. An Edwards-Venn diagram was used to present patients' numbers and success rates using topical anti-glaucoma medications based on their ingredients. The area under the receiver operating characteristic curve (AUROC) was calculated to compare the effects of several factors on the EDCR success rate. Statistical significance was set at $p < 0.05$.

3. Results

During the study period, EDCR was performed on 30 eyes of 30 patients receiving anti-glaucoma medication. A total of 120 patients were enrolled in this study, including 30 in the anti-glaucoma medication group and 90 age- and sex-matched controls. The demographic characteristics of the patients are shown in Table 1.

Table 1. Demographics of the patients.

Characteristics	Anti-Glaucoma Medication Group ($n = 30$)	Control Group ($n = 90$)	p-Value
Age (years ± SD)	68.1 ± 9.9	68.1 ± 8.5	0.967 *
Gender (n, %)			
Male	7 (23.3)	21 (23.3)	0.999 †
Female	23 (76.7)	69 (76.7)	
DM	8 (26.7)	10 (11.1)	0.072 ‡
HTN	15 (50.0)	30 (33.3)	0.102 †
Laterality (right, %)	12 (40.0)	51 (56.7)	0.113 †

SD = standard deviation; DM = diabetic mellitus; HTN = hypertension. * Independent t-test, † Chi-square test, ‡ Fisher's exact test.

The mean age was 68.1 years, and the female-to-male ratio was 3.3:1. No statistically significant differences were observed in age, sex, laterality, or underlying systemic diseases between the groups. In this study, patients were administered various combinations of anti-glaucoma ingredients. Consequently, we analyzed the number of patients and EDCR success rates of the four overlapping ingredients using an Edwards-Venn diagram (Figure 1). Six months after surgery, the success rates were 97.8% in the control group and 86.7% in the anti-glaucoma medication group ($p = 0.034$). When analyzed based on the glaucoma types, the success rates for the control group, normal tension glaucoma, primary open-angle glaucoma, pseudoexfoliation glaucoma (PXF), and chronic angle-closure glaucoma (CACG) were 97.8% (88/90), 90.0% (10/11), 85.7% (12/14), 100.0% (2/2), and 66.7% (2/3) ($p = 0.035$). However, the CACG group and the PXF group each consisted of only two patients. Also, in the post-hoc analysis, the CACG group did not exhibit statistical significance ($p = 0.360$). When analyzed based on the severity of glaucoma according to mean deviation in the visual field, the success rates for early glaucoma, moderate glaucoma, and severe glaucoma were 88.9% (8/9), 100.0% (8/8), and 76.9% (10/13) ($p = 0.311$).

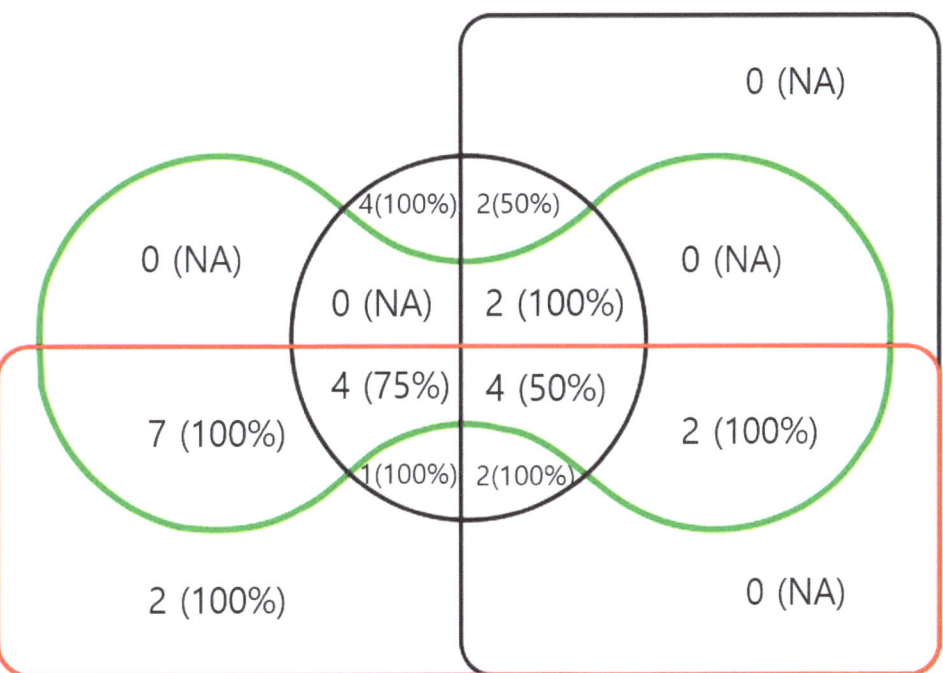

Figure 1. The Edwards-Venn diagram shows the number and the success rates (within parentheses) of patients using anti-glaucoma medication according to ingredients. Black box: alpha agonists. Red box: beta-blockers. Black circle: prostaglandin analogs. Green curve: carbonic anhydrase inhibitors. NA: not assessed.

Six months after surgery, the success rates were 97.8% (control group), 86.4% (beta-blockers), 75.0% (alpha-agonists), 84.2% (carbonic anhydrase inhibitors [CAI]), and 78.9% (prostaglandin [PG] analogs). Using univariate logistic regression analysis, alpha-agonists (odds ratio [OR], 0.086; 95% confidence interval [CI], 0.015–0.488, $p = 0.006$), CAI (OR, 0.163; 95% CI, 0.030–0.881, $p = 0.035$), and PG (OR, 0.076; 95% CI, 0.013–0.450, $p = 0.005$) were found to be negative risk factors for EDCR success rate (Table 2). Multivariate backward elimination was performed to analyze the ingredients that had the greatest impact on the EDCR success rate among the four ingredients of the anti-glaucoma medication. Multivariate logistic regression analysis revealed that PGs were the most influential risk factor for EDCR success among the anti-glaucoma medication ingredients (OR, 0.076; 95% CI, 0.013–0.450; p = 0.005). When analyzed according to subtypes of PG, the success rates for the control group, latanoprost, tafluprost, bimatoprost, and travoprost were 97.8% (88/90), 70.0 (7/10), 100.0% (5/5), 100.0% (2/2), and 50.0% (1/2) (p = 0.005). The success rates decreased in the latanoprost and travoprost group. However, in the post-hoc analysis, neither group exhibited statistical significance (p = 0.999 and p = 0.580), respectively.

Table 2. Risk factors affecting the success rate of EDCR based on anti-glaucoma medication ingredients.

	Univariate			Multivariate		
	B	OR (95% CI)	p-Value *	B	OR (95% CI)	p-Value *
Beta-blockers	−1.609	0.200 (0.037–1.067)	0.060			
Alpha agonists	−2.457	0.086 (0.015–0.488)	0.006			
Carbonic anhydrase inhibitors	−1.812	0.163 (0.030–0.881)	0.035			
Prostaglandin analogs	−2.580	0.076 (0.013–0.450)	0.005	−2.580	0.076 (0.013–0.450)	0.005

EDCR = endoscopic dacryocystorhinostomy; OR = odds ratio; CI = confidence interval; * Logistic regression analysis.

We also analyzed the success rates according to the number of anti-glaucoma medication ingredients. Success rates were compared when one, two, three, and all four drug ingredients were used. The success rates were 97.8% (control), 100.0% (one ingredient), 90.0% (two ingredients), 90.0% (three ingredients), and 50.0% (all four ingredients) (p = 0.010). The success rate of patients, including all four anti-glaucoma medication ingredients, was also statistically significant in the post-hoc analysis (p = 0.008) (Table 3).

Table 3. Comparisons of EDCR success rates according to anti-glaucoma medication ingredients.

	Control Group (n = 90)	One Ingredient (n = 6)	Two Ingredients (n = 10)	Three Ingredients (n = 10)	Four Ingredients (n = 4)	p-Value
EDCR Success rates	88 (97.8%)	6 (100%)	9 (90.0%)	9 (90.0%)	2 (50.0%)	0.010 ‡
Post-hoc analysis		0.999 ‡	0.273 ‡	0.273 ‡	0.008 ‡	

EDCR = endoscopic dacryocystorhinostomy; ‡ Fisher's exact test.

The success rates were also compared according to the duration of anti-glaucoma medication use. The success rates were 97.8% (control group), 91.7% (duration < 12 months), 100.0% (12–24 months), and 76.9% (>24 months) (p = 0.019). In the group of patients who used anti-glaucoma medication for >24 months, the success rate was significantly different among the three groups (p = 0.019). The post-hoc analysis yielded a p-value of 0.083, slightly higher than the significance level of 0.05 (Table 4).

Table 4. Comparisons of EDCR success rates according to the duration of anti-glaucoma medication use in months.

	Control Group (n = 90)	≤12 Months (n = 12)	12–24 Months (n = 5)	>24 Months (n = 13)	p-Value
EDCR success rates	88 (97.8%)	11 (91.7)	5 (100.0)	10 (76.9)	0.019 ‡
Post-hoc analysis		0.316 ‡	0.999 ‡	0.083 ‡	

EDCR = endoscopic dacryocystorhinostomy; ‡ Fisher's exact test.

When the number of drug ingredients was multiplied by the duration in months, the median value was 69. The anti-glaucoma medication group was divided into two groups based on median values. The success rates were 97.8% (control group), 93.3% (group 1, ≤69), and 80.0% (Group 2, >69). The EDCR success rate in Group 2 was significantly decreased (p = 0.022). The post-hoc analysis yielded a p-value of 0.061, slightly higher than the significance level of 0.05 (Table 5).

Table 5. Comparisons of the success rates of EDCR based on the product of ingredient numbers multiplied by duration in months.

	Control Group (n = 90)	Group 1 (≤69) (n = 15)	Group 2 (>69) (n = 15)	p-Value
EDCR success rates	88 (97.8%)	14 (93.3)	12 (80.0)	0.022 ‡
Post-hoc analysis		0.746 ‡	0.061 ‡	

EDCR = endoscopic dacryocystorhinostomy; ‡ Fisher's exact test.

Univariate logistic regression analysis showed that the number of anti-glaucoma medications (OR, 0.437; 95% CI, 0.247–0.772, $p = 0.004$), duration of anti-glaucoma medication (OR, 0.981; 95% CI, 0.964–0.997, $p = 0.020$), and the product of ingredient numbers multiplied by duration in months (OR, 0.991; 95% CI, 0.983–0.997, $p = 0.009$) were negative risk factors for EDCR success rate. Multivariate backward elimination was employed to analyze the risk factors that had the greatest influence on the EDCR success rate. Multivariate logistic regression analysis indicated that the number of anti-glaucoma medications was the only risk factor for EDCR success rate (OR, 0.437; 95% CI, 0.247–0.772; $p = 0.004$) (Table 6).

Table 6. Univariate and multivariate logistic regression analyses for success rate of EDCR.

	B	Univariate OR (95% CI)	p-Value *	B	Multivariate OR (95% CI)	p-Value *
Age	−0.004	0.996 (0.907–1.094)	0.941			
Sex	−0.477	0.621 (0.108–3.577)	0.594			
DM	−0.132	0.876 (0.096–7.972)	0.907			
HTN	−0.539	0.583 (0.113–3.022)	0.521			
Mean deviation of VF	0.028	1.028 (0.911–1.160)	0.654			
Number of glaucoma medication	−0.829	0.437 (0.247–0.772)	0.004	−0.829	0.437 (0.247–0.772)	0.004
Duration of glaucoma medication	−0.020	0.981 (0.964–0.997)	0.020			
Product of ingredient numbers multiplied by duration in months	−0.010	0.991 (0.983–0.997)	0.009			

EDCR = endoscopic dacryocystorhinostomy; OR = odds ratio; DM = diabetic mellitus; HTN = hypertension; VF = visual field; * Logistic regression analysis.

The receiver operating characteristic curve (ROC) curve of the number of anti-glaucoma medications showed a limited area under the ROC curve (AUC) of 0.760 (95% CI, 0.674–0.833, $p = 0.031$), with a sensitivity of 82.5% and a specificity of 66.7%. The ROC curves for the duration of anti-glaucoma medication use (AUC = 0.741; 95% CI, 0.653–0.817; $p = 0.037$) and the product of ingredient number multiplied by duration (AUC = 0.752; 95% CI, 0.665–0.826; $p = 0.033$) were similar. However, the AUC of the number of anti-glaucoma medications was higher than that of the other two variables (Figure 2).

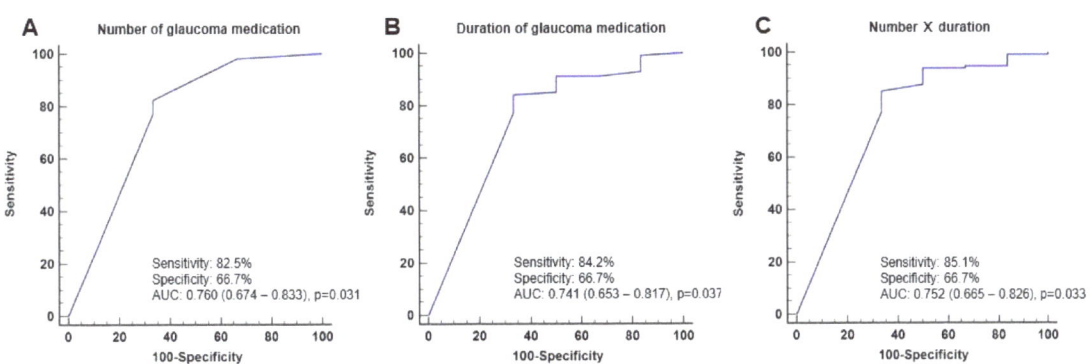

Figure 2. The ROC curves showing the success rates of endoscopic dacryocystorhinostomy accor–ing to risk factors. The ROC curves according to (A) number of glaucoma medication, (B) duration of glaucoma medication, and (C) the product of ingredient number multiplied by duration.

4. Discussion

According to previous studies, 5–23% [2–4] of patients were receiving anti-glaucoma treatment when lacrimal drainage system obstruction was being diagnosed. In our study of 795 patients with NLDO, 30 (3.8%) used topical anti-glaucoma medications during EDCR surgery. Some studies have reported that anti-glaucoma medications induce inflammatory and fibrotic changes on the conjunctival surface. Likewise, they may induce inflammation and fibrosis in the epithelium and subepithelial tissue of the lacrimal drainage system, causing NLDO [4,13,14]. Furthermore, previous studies have reported that topical anti-glaucoma medications may exaggerate the scarring response in the mucosa of the lacrimal drainage system and affect the success rate of EDCR [3,9]. Di Maria et al. [9] hypothesized that the toxicity of anti-glaucoma medications induces fibrosis in the mucous membranes of the lacrimal system. Mandel et al. [3] demonstrated that nasal endoscopy in failed DCR surgery in patients treated with anti-glaucoma medications showed mucosal scarring at the anastomosis site. Our results also aligned with these hypotheses, as the success rate was low in the anti-glaucoma medication group ($p = 0.034$). We also thought there might be a difference in EDCR success rates depending on the glaucoma types or severity, but no significant difference was found. Although the success rate was relatively low in the CACG group (66.7%) and patients with severe visual field defects (76.9%), there was no statistical significance. Because the number of subjects in each group is small, detailed analysis is challenging, so a large-scale study is needed.

We aimed to exclude patients with severe deformities in the osteomeatal complex that could potentially decrease the success rate of DCR and ensure a representative sample of NLDO by obtaining orbital CT scans. The preoperative imaging helps in recognizing the bony anatomy surrounding the lacrimal outflow system, the mucous membranes, normal anatomic variants, sinusitis, tumors, and previous trauma [15]. The correlation between nasal septal deviation, sinusitis, and structural abnormalities of the sinonasal cavity and NLDO has been studied, but the results are still inconclusive [16]. Therefore, we did not exclude all minor anatomic variants, but we tried to exclude severe scar formation or synechia resulting from trauma, tumors, or previous operations, as they could potentially contribute to the failure of DCR.

Several studies have reported that certain ingredients of topical anti-glaucoma medications might have a greater effect on epiphora; however, a unified opinion has not been established. Although Oritz-Basso et al. [13] showed no evidence that any particular ingredient of an anti-glaucoma medication carries a higher risk of NLDO, other studies have indicated that specific ingredients of anti-glaucoma medications carry a higher risk. The ingredients were diverse, including timolol [4], dorzolamide [14], CAI [3], and PGs [9]; however, their hypothesis consistently suggested that anti-glaucoma medication ingredients influence the distal excretory lacrimal mucosa, leading to fibrosis. However, the precise mechanisms underlying inflammation and fibrosis remain unclear. In our study, alpha agonists, CAIs, and PGs were negative risk factors for the EDCR success rate. And PGs were the most influential risk factor for the EDCR success rate among glaucoma medication ingredients. Our results support the relationship between the use of topical PGs and fibrosis in NLD. Unlike other glaucoma medications, PG has generally been associated with intraocular inflammation because it can potentially induce further inflammatory responses. Therefore, the use of PG is recommended with caution in patients with an inflammatory history such as uveitis, herpes keratitis, and inflammatory glaucoma [17]. PGs likely trigger chronic inflammation by regulating immune cells and crosstalking with cytokines [18]. Endogenous PGs have a role in inflammatory mediation in the eyes and are considered a potent proinflammatory agent responsible for uveitis or cystoid macular edema [19]. The exact cause-and-effect relationship between PG-inducing exacerbations of uveitis or CME has not been elucidated. However, in animal studies, ocular inflammation was induced when a large amount of PG was administered to rabbit eyes [20], and there are numerous case reports supporting this. It can be inferred that these inflammatory mechanisms can also affect the NLD mucosa. Therefore, given the observed decreased success rate of EDCR in the PG group within this study, surgeons might contemplate switching preoperative anti-glaucoma medications to non-PG medications for concurrent glaucoma patients requiring DCR surgery.

We also hypothesized that the subtypes of PG might have different effects on the eyes. We analyzed the success rate of PG subtypes by classifying them into latanoprost, tafluprost, bimatoprost, and travoprost. However, due to the small patient numbers in each group, significant effects were not found. The adverse effects of PG, such as eyelid pigmentation, iris pigmentation, hypertrichosis around the eye, and deepening of the upper eyelid sulcus, are referred to as prostaglandin-associated periorbitopathy (PAP). Also, PAP was reported to be more frequent and severe in the bimatoprost group compared with other PG subtypes [21,22]. As reported by pharmacological studies, bimatoprost accumulates in higher concentrations in eyelid tissues than in the aqueous humor, iris, and ciliary body [23]. Therefore, bimatoprost might have the most negative impact on the eyelid compared with other PG subtypes. In contrast, an in vitro study revealed that bimatoprost exhibited lower cytotoxicity in conjunctiva-derived epithelial cells when compared with other PG subtypes [24]. Guenon et al. [24] reported that in commercial preparations, bimatoprost contains less benzalkonium chloride (BAK) than travoprost and latanoprost. Since ocular surface toxicity was associated with the concentration of the preservative BAK, bimatoprost showed lower cytotoxicity. Bimatoprost induced more side effects in the eyelid compared with other PGs; however, it exhibited lower toxicity in the conjunctiva. It is not known what side effects PG subtypes may induce in the NLD, and additional research is needed.

In addition to active ingredients, the preservatives in anti-glaucoma medications are also an issue. Topical anti-glaucoma medications are composed of active ingredients, preservatives, and excipients and are known to be associated with inflammatory and fibrotic changes on the ocular surface [5–8]. In particular, preservatives in anti-glaucoma medications destabilize bacterial cell membranes and have the same effect on normal corneal and conjunctival cells, thereby causing OSD [8]. OSD occurred more frequently in patients with increased glaucoma severity and was associated with higher exposure to BAK. A daily dose of BAK of more than three drops was an independent predictor of the OSD index score [25]. Although they did not directly compare preservative-containing and preservative-free glaucoma medications, several studies have suggested that active ingredients or preservatives in anti-glaucoma medications may contribute to the development of NLDO, similar to their role in inducing OSD [9,13]. However, Mandel et al. [3] reported no significant difference in the success rate of primary DCR between patients treated with preserved and those treated with non-preserved anti-glaucoma medications. In our study, all patients with glaucoma used preservative-containing eye drops. Therefore, assessing the impact of preservatives or excipients was impossible. However, it might be more advantageous to analyze the effects of active ingredients on NLD. Further studies are needed to investigate the potential effects of preservatives and excipients on the development of NLDO and the success rates of DCR. In our study, as it appeared that PG showed significant relevance to the success rate of DCR, it is necessary to compare the success rates of DCR among the control group, the non-preserved PG group, and the preserved PG group. Furthermore, when patients receiving anti-glaucoma treatment require DCR surgery, surgeons should consider switching from preservative-containing anti-glaucoma medications to preservative-free anti-glaucoma medications.

The cumulative dosage should also be considered, as glaucoma requires continuous eye-drop management. Variables such as the number of drugs, duration of use, and their combinations may contribute to cumulative effects. This study examined the success rate of EDCR regarding the number, duration, and cumulative effects of anti-glaucoma medications.

Seider et al. [4] reported that the number of topical anti-glaucoma medications was higher in the NLDO group than in the control group (1.58 vs. 0.73, $p = 0.002$). However, Ortiz-Basso et al. [13] reported that the proportion of patients using more than two anti-glaucoma medications was not higher in the NLDO group (67% vs. 62%, $p = 0.491$). In our study, patients treated with all four anti-glaucoma ingredients exhibited a decreased EDCR success rate ($p = 0.008$). However, the group of patients using all four anti-glaucoma ingredients consisted of only four patients. Therefore, the small number of patients may have introduced a bias. In the logistic regression analysis, the number of anti-glaucoma medications was the most relevant risk factor among the variables. We assumed the number of anti-glaucoma medications had the most prominent cumulative effect. In our study, we observed a reduced success rate when PGs were used. However, because PGs are the most commonly used first-line treatment, they are frequently part of the regimen for patients using multiple anti-glaucoma medications. Therefore, it is challenging to determine whether the reduced success rate is due to the presence of PGs or the cumulative effects of multiple eye drop ingredients.

The occurrence of NLDO after using anti-glaucoma medications has been mentioned as an idiosyncratic reaction in short-term use cases and a potential cumulative effect in long-term use cases; however, no statistically significant evidence has been provided [14]. In our study, patients using eye drops for >24 months showed a decreased EDCR success rate ($p = 0.019$). We assumed a cumulative effect of long-term use of anti-glaucoma medications.

According to our results, the number of ingredients and the duration of use contributed to a decrease in the EDCR surgical success rate. The authors observed a correlation between the number of ingredients and the duration of use, similar to the pack-year analysis in smokers. Consequently, we reanalyzed the product of these two factors as a single variable. The patients were divided into two groups based on the median value of the product obtained by multiplying the number of ingredients by the number of months of use. The success rate of EDCR was significantly decreased in Group 2 (>69) ($p = 0.022$). Although the group using anti-glaucoma medication for > 24 months and Group 2 (>69) were both statistically significant ($p = 0.019$ and $p = 0.022$, respectively), the post-hoc p-values were 0.083 and 0.061, respectively, which were slightly higher than the significant p-value of 0.05. However, it could be considered a borderline value in post-hoc analysis, indicating a potential tendency toward a decrease in the success rate of EDCR. When there are significant p-values implying overall differences among groups, post-hoc analysis is needed to identify which groups differ from each other. It is anticipated that with an increase in the number of patients, the p-values in post-hoc analysis might also become more evident. Although our study included more patients than previous studies, the number of patients with glaucoma was still insufficient for analyzing risk factors. Therefore, the small number of patients may have introduced bias. Considering that the post-hoc p-value was slightly higher than the significance level of 0.05, it may be necessary to confirm the significance by analyzing a larger number of patients.

We multiplied the number of drug ingredients by the duration in months to analyze the cumulative effects. AUROC was evaluated to compare which factor is more related to EDCR success rates. The ROC curves and AUC indicated similar relevance among the number of anti-glaucoma medication ingredients, duration of medication, and product of the number of drug ingredients multiplied by duration in months. The AUC of the number of anti-glaucoma medications was higher than that of the other two variables. Although the product of the number of drug ingredients multiplied by duration in months did not show better results than the other two variables in AUROC, this is the first study to analyze the cumulative effect of anti-glaucoma medications. Further discussion on appropriate methods for measuring cumulative effects is needed.

A limitation of our study is that all patients received topical anti-glaucoma medications containing preservatives, which could affect the success rate. Accurately excluding the effects of preservatives from the success rate of EDCR was challenging. In addition, the group using anti-glaucoma medications for more than 24 months and Group 2 (>69) were both statistically significant but not in the post-hoc analysis. The limitation of our study can be attributed to its relatively small sample size. Further prospective studies with larger sample sizes are required to confirm our findings.

In conclusion, the success rate of EDCR surgery decreased in patients receiving anti-glaucoma medications. PG-containing eye drops, a higher number of ingredients, a longer duration of use, and the cumulative effect of both the number and duration contributed to a decrease in the surgical success rate. A higher number of drug ingredients was the most influential factor among the variables. Therefore, when performing EDCR on patients using topical anti-glaucoma medications, surgeons should inform patients about the possibility of increased recurrence rates after EDCR surgery.

Author Contributions: Design and execution of the study, S.E.L. and S.B.L.; collection of data, S.E.L. and S.O.; analysis and interpretation of data, S.E.L., H.B.L., K.L. and S.B.L.; writing the article, S.E.L. and S.B.L.; critical revision of the article, S.E.L. and S.B.L.; final approval of the article S.E.L., H.B.L., S.O., K.L. and S.B.L. All authors have read and agreed to the published version of the manuscript.

Funding: This research received no external funding.

Institutional Review Board Statement: The study was conducted according to the guidelines of the Declaration of Helsinki and approved by the Institutional Review Board of Chungnam National University Hospital. (IRB no. 2023-03-016, date of approval: 21 March 2023).

Informed Consent Statement: Patient consent was waived due to the retrospective nature of the study.

Data Availability Statement: Data supporting the findings of the current study are available from the corresponding author on reasonable request.

Conflicts of Interest: The authors declare no conflicts of interest.

References

1. Kashkouli, M.B.; Sadeghipour, A.; Kaghazkanani, R.; Bayat, A.; Pakdel, F.; Aghai, G.H. Pathogenesis of primary acquired nasolacrimal duct obstruction. *Orbit* **2010**, *29*, 11–15. [CrossRef] [PubMed]
2. Woog, J.J. The incidence of symptomatic acquired lacrimal outflow obstruction among residents of Olmsted County, Minnesota, 1976-2000 (an American Ophthalmological Society thesis). *Trans. Am. Ophthalmol. Soc.* **2007**, *105*, 649–666. [PubMed]
3. Mandal, P.; Ahluwalia, H. Do topical ocular antihypertensives affect Dacryocystorhinostomy outcomes: The Coventry experience. *Eye* **2022**, *36*, 135–139. [CrossRef] [PubMed]
4. Seider, N.; Miller, B.; Beiran, I. Topical glaucoma therapy as a risk factor for nasolacrimal duct obstruction. *Am. J. Ophthalmol.* **2008**, *145*, 120–123. [CrossRef] [PubMed]
5. Ruangvaravate, N.; Prabhasawat, P.; Vachirasakchai, V.; Tantimala, R. High Prevalence of Ocular Surface Disease among Glaucoma Patients in Thailand. *J. Ocul. Pharmacol. Ther.* **2018**, *34*, 387–394. [CrossRef]
6. Aydin Kurna, S.; Acikgoz, S.; Altun, A.; Ozbay, N.; Sengor, T.; Olcaysu, O.O. The effects of topical antiglaucoma drugs as monotherapy on the ocular surface: A prospective study. *J. Ophthalmol.* **2014**, *2014*, 460483. [CrossRef]
7. Ruangvaravate, N.; Choojun, K.; Srikulsasitorn, B.; Chokboonpiem, J.; Asanatong, D.; Trakanwitthayarak, S. Ocular Surface Changes After Switching from Other Prostaglandins to Tafluprost and Preservative-Free Tafluprost in Glaucoma Patients. *Clin. Ophthalmol.* **2020**, *14*, 3109–3119. [CrossRef]
8. Inoue, K. Managing adverse effects of glaucoma medications. *Clin. Ophthalmol.* **2014**, *8*, 903–913. [CrossRef]
9. Di Maria, A.; Tredici, C.; Cozzupoli, G.M.; Vinciguerra, P.; Confalonieri, F. Effects of prostaglandin analogues on epiphora persistence after EN-DCR: A hypothesis-generating study. *Eur. J. Ophthalmol.* **2023**, *33*, 182–187. [CrossRef]
10. Katz, J.; Sommer, A.; Gaasterland, D.E.; Anderson, D.R. Comparison of analytic algorithms for detecting glaucomatous visual field loss. *Arch. Ophthalmol.* **1991**, *109*, 1684–1689. [CrossRef]
11. Feuer, W.J.; Anderson, D.R. Static threshold asymmetry in early glaucomatous visual field loss. *Ophthalmology* **1989**, *96*, 1285–1297. [CrossRef] [PubMed]
12. Lee, N.H.; Park, K.S.; Lee, H.M.; Kim, J.Y.; Kim, C.S.; Kim, K.N. Using the Thickness Map from Macular Ganglion Cell Analysis to Differentiate Retinal Vein Occlusion from Glaucoma. *J. Clin. Med.* **2020**, *9*, 3294. [CrossRef]
13. Ortiz-Basso, T.; Galmarini, A.; Vigo, R.L.; Gonzalez-Barlatay, J.M.; Premoli, E.J. The relationship between topical anti-glaucoma medications and the development of lacrimal drainage system obstruction. *Arq. Bras. Oftalmol.* **2018**, *81*, 490–493. [CrossRef]
14. Kashkouli, M.B.; Rezaee, R.; Nilforoushan, N.; Salimi, S.; Foroutan, A.; Naseripour, M. Topical antiglaucoma medications and lacrimal drainage system obstruction. *Ophthalmic Plast. Reconstr. Surg.* **2008**, *24*, 172–175. [CrossRef]
15. Medghalchi, A.; Alizadeh, Y.; Dourandeesh, M.; Fallah Arzpeima, S.; Soltani Moghadami, R.; Akbari, M.; Khadem, S.; Kazem-nezhad Leyli, E. Preoperative orbital CT scan findings in patients with nasolacrimal duct obstruction and its impact on surgical planning. *J. Kerman Univ. Med. Sci.* **2023**, *30*, 248–252. [CrossRef]
16. Su, P.Y.; Wang, J.K.; Chang, S.W. Computed Tomography Morphology of Affected versus Unaffected Sides in Patients with Unilateral Primary Acquired Nasolacrimal Duct Obstruction. *J. Clin. Med.* **2023**, *12*, 340. [CrossRef]

17. Kroll, D.M.; Schuman, J.S. Reactivation of herpes simplex virus keratitis after initiating bimatoprost treatment for glaucoma. *Am. J. Ophthalmol.* **2002**, *133*, 401–403. [CrossRef]
18. Yao, C.; Narumiya, S. Prostaglandin-cytokine crosstalk in chronic inflammation. *Br. J. Pharmacol.* **2019**, *176*, 337–354. [CrossRef]
19. Hu, J.; Vu, J.T.; Hong, B.; Gottlieb, C. Uveitis and cystoid macular oedema secondary to topical prostaglandin analogue use in ocular hypertension and open angle glaucoma. *Br. J. Ophthalmol.* **2020**, *104*, 1040–1044. [CrossRef]
20. Eakins, K.E. Prostaglandin and non-prostaglandin mediated breeakdown of the blood-aqueous barrier. *Exp Eye Res.* **1977**, *25*, 483–498. [CrossRef]
21. Inoue, K.; Shiokawa, M.; Higa, R.; Sugahara, M.; Soga, T.; Wakakura, M.; Tomita, G. Adverse periocular reactions to five types of prostaglandin analogs. *Eye* **2012**, *26*, 1465–1472. [CrossRef] [PubMed]
22. Kucukevcilioglu, M.; Bayer, A.; Uysal, Y.; Altinsoy, H.I. Prostaglandin associated periorbitopathy in patients using bimatoprost, latanoprost and travoprost. *Clin. Exp. Ophthalmol.* **2014**, *42*, 126–131. [CrossRef] [PubMed]
23. Woodward, D.F.; Krauss, A.-P.; Chen, J.; Liang, Y.; Li, C.; Protzman, C.E.; Bogardus, A.; Chen, R.; Kedzie, K.M.; Krauss, H.A.; et al. Pharmacological characterization of a novel antiglaucoma agent, Bimatoprost (AGN 192024). *J. Pharmacol. Exp. Ther.* **2003**, *305*, 772–785. [CrossRef] [PubMed]
24. Guenoun, J.-M.; Baudouin, C.; Rat, P.; Pauly, A.; Warnet, J.-M.; Brignole-Baudouin, F. In Vitro Study of Inflammatory Potential and Toxicity Profile of Latanoprost, Travoprost, and Bimatoprost in Conjunctiva-Derived Epithelial Cells. *Investig. Ophthalmol. Vis. Sci.* **2005**, *46*, 2444–2450. [CrossRef]
25. Skalicky, S.E.; Goldberg, I.; McCluskey, P. Ocular surface disease and quality of life in patients with glaucoma. *Am. J. Ophthalmol.* **2012**, *153*, 1–9.e2. [CrossRef]

Disclaimer/Publisher's Note: The statements, opinions and data contained in all publications are solely those of the individual author(s) and contributor(s) and not of MDPI and/or the editor(s). MDPI and/or the editor(s) disclaim responsibility for any injury to people or property resulting from any ideas, methods, instructions or products referred to in the content.

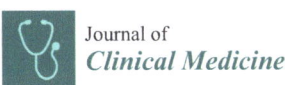

Article

Comparison of Outcomes of Silicone Tube Intubation with or without Dacryoendoscopy for the Treatment of Congenital Nasolacrimal Duct Obstruction

Doah Kim and Helen Lew *

Department of Ophthalmology, CHA Bundang Medical Center, CHA University, Seongnam 13496, Republic of Korea; a216015@chamc.co.kr
* Correspondence: eye@cha.ac.kr; Tel./Fax: +82-31-780-5330

Abstract: In this retrospective study, we compared and analyzed two groups of patients who underwent silicone tube intubation (STI) to treat congenital nasolacrimal duct obstruction (CNDO). We employed dacryoendoscopy to visualize the lacrimal pathways of one group. In total, 85 eyes of 69 patients were included (52 of 41 patients in the non-dacryoendoscopy and 33 eyes of 28 patients in the dacryoendoscopy group). Clinical characteristics, dacryoendoscopic findings, and surgical outcomes were evaluated. The overall STI success rate was 91.8%, and the success rate was significantly higher in the dacryoendoscopy versus non-dacryoendoscopy group (97.0% and 88.5%, respectively). For patients < 36 months of age, the success rate was 100% (23 eyes). All patients with Hasner valve membranous obstructions were younger than 36 months and had structural obstructions of the lacrimal drainage system (LDS) ($p = 0.04$). However, in patients lacking Hasner valve obstructions, LDS secretory (50.0%) and structural (50%) obstructions occurred at similar rates, which did not vary by age. Dacryoendoscopy-assisted STI enhanced the therapeutic efficacy of CNDO and identified diverse CNDO etiologies beyond Hasner valve obstructions. These findings emphasize the potential advantages of dacryoendoscopy in surgical treatment for CNDO patients.

Keywords: congenital nasolacrimal duct obstruction; dacryoendoscpy; silicone tube intubation

1. Introduction

Congenital nasolacrimal duct obstruction (CNDO) is the most common cause of childhood epiphora [1] and is typically caused by obstruction of the Hasner valve at the end of the nasolacrimal duct [2,3]. The spontaneous CNDO resolution rate in the first year of life is in the range of 62.8–95.0% [4–8]. CNDO treatment is stepwise in nature [9]. In infants younger than 6 months, management is conservative (lacrimal sac massage). Subsequently, probing is the first-line invasive treatment [8,10]. The initial probing success rate is 87.2% in children aged 2 weeks to 41 months, but decreases thereafter [11]. If probing is ineffective, silicone tube intubation (STI) is possible; the success rate is 62–100% [12–14].

Dacryoendoscopy enables direct CNDO visualization, thus revealing the various pathologies [8]. Dacryoendoscopy allows analysis of membranous obstructions of the Hasner valve, which are the most common cause of NDO; the obstructions have various morphologies. Obstructions at the distal end of the Hasner valve are divided into simple and complicated types. The simple type is a thin blockage that is readily penetrated; the complicated type involves stenosis or fibrosis [14]. However, Nishi et al. reported that only 15.4% of lower nasolacrimal fibroses were revealed by dacryoendoscopy in CNDO children who failed probing [13]. Lacrimal duct mucosal injuries were identified in 69.2% of such children; dacryoendoscopy-assisted incision of the Hasner valve membrane under nasal endoscopic guidance was associated with a high success rate [15]. Although conventional STI (without dacryoendoscopy) also has a high success rate, the various complications include the creation of false passages, punctum erosion, and the formation of pyogenic

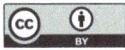

granulomas [6,13]. Thus, dacryoendoscopy is being increasingly used for lacrimal drainage system (LDS) examination and treatment [13]. Previously, we reported a higher success rate of dacryoendoscopy-assisted STI compared to cases without dacryoendoscopy in patients with primary acquired nasolacrimal duct obstruction [16]. However, few studies have explored whether the use of dacryoendoscopy during STI for CNDO children enhances treatment success. Also, no single-center, single-surgeon study has determined whether dacryoendoscopy improves STI outcomes, which we investigate herein. Therefore, we aimed to identify the best surgical technique. Additionally, we analyzed the internal LDS morphology and that of the Hasner valve at the distal end of the lacrimal duct.

2. Materials and Methods

The study and the data collection protocol were approved by the Institutional Review Board of CHA Bundang Medical Center, Seongnam, Republic of Korea (approval no. 2023-09-035, approval date 31 October 2023). The study adhered to the tenets of the Declaration of Helsinki. Informed consent was obtained from all parents or guardians prior to patient enrolment.

2.1. Subjects

We retrospectively reviewed the medical records of CNDO patients who underwent STI at the CHA Bundang Medical Center from January 2013 to January 2022. We included children aged $\geq$ 12 months, or who had failed probing at least once when aged $\leq$ 12 months. We explained the stepwise treatment for CNDO to the parents of all subjects, and STI was performed for those who consented to surgical treatment. Before the surgery, we explained the purpose, procedure, and potential complications to the parents of all subjects, and informed consent was obtained. All subjects were divided into dacryoendoscopy and non-dacryoendoscopy groups. The conventional group (STI without dacryoendoscopy) included 52 eyes of 41 patients aged 9–117 months treated from January 2013 to July 2016. Among the patients aged < 12 months, one aged 9 months had previously undergone (unsuccessful) probing 3 times, and 38 eyes belonged to subjects aged < 36 months. The dacryoendoscopy-assisted STI group comprised 33 eyes of 28 patients aged 11–123 months treated from August 2016 to January 2022. Two of these patients were <12 months of age (both aged 11 months), and they had both previously undergone unsuccessful probing twice; twenty-three eyes belonged to subjects < 36 months of age. We diagnosed clinical CNDO when epiphora or "sticky eye" was apparent. We excluded children with congenital anomalies such as Down syndrome, as well as those who did not undergo preoperative dacryoscintigraphy (DSG) and those who were lost to follow-up. At the first follow-up visit 1 week post surgery, signs and symptoms were assessed. Surgical success was defined as either the complete resolution of previous signs and symptoms or a successful irrigation test result; follow-up continued for 3 months after extubation. Worsening of signs and symptoms following successful intubation was considered surgical failure.

2.2. Transcanalicular Dacryoplasty

From August 2016, we utilized a dacryoendoscope (FT-203F; Fibertech Co., Tokyo, Japan), which possessed the following specifications: probe outer diameter of 0.6 mm, field of view of 70°, 6000 image elements, and an observation depth ranging from 1 to 10 mm. A sheath (Angio catheter, Daewon, Seoul, Republic of Korea) was used to cover and dilate the lumen, with the possibility of movement within the LDS. The nasal endoscope (7208CA; Karl Strotz, Tuttlingen, Germany) had a probe outer diameter of 2.7 mm, a view angle direction of 0°, and 410,000 image elements. All cases were conducted under general anesthesia, and all STI was performed using both dacryoendoscopy and nasal endoscopy. After a subconjunctival injection of 2.0 mL lidocaine 2% with a 30-G needle, we dilated the upper and lower lacrimal punctum with a punctal dilator and inserted the dacryoendoscope through them. The dacryoendoscopy was slowly moved toward the canaliculus, and gently forward to the lacrimal sac. For clear viewing of the lumen, saline was injected through the water channel. On reaching the lacrimal sac, we held the dacryoendoscopy upright and pushed it forward to the lacrimal duct while visually guided by the dacryoendoscopy. Using dacryoendoscopy, we examined the inside of the LDS to determine the level and pattern of obstruction. When the dacryoendoscope passed through the LDS, the nasal endoscope provided the morphological findings of the distal end of the inferior meatus, also known as Hasner's valve. A bicanalicular silicone tube with a 0.6 mm diameter (YWL84; E&I Tech, Kyungki-do, Republic of Korea) was inserted while under visual guidance. The tube was then retrieved, and both ends were locked and stabilized under the inferior turbinate. All surgical treatments, STI, and dacryoendoscopy examinations were performed by a single surgeon (H.L.).

2.3. Classification of Dacryoendoscopic Findings

The endoscopic findings of CNDO were analyzed based on two criteria: findings observed at both the end of the lacrimal duct, including Hasner's valve and the LDS. First, the morphology of Hasner's valve was classified into two types: simple and complicated (fibrosis, stenosis). The simple type was defined as a thin blockage of the Hasner's valve membrane that could be easily perforated without resistance. The complicated type included fibrosis, which was characterized by a dense fibrous blockage at the end of Hasner's valve, and stenosis, which was defined as a structural narrowing that caused resistance around Hasner's valve and resulted in a diameter of the end that was smaller than that of the dacryoendoscope (0.6 mm). The presence of a membrane at the Hasner's valve was defined as cases with very thick membranes that were clearly visible on dacryoendoscopy and nasal endoscopy. Second, throughout the LDS, the pattern of obstruction was classified into two subtypes: the secretory type, such as mucus or dacryolith, and the structural type, such as stenosis or membrane.

2.4. Statistical Analysis

IBM SPSS software (ver. 23.0; IBM Corp., Armonk, NY, USA) was used for all statistical analyses. Parametric and non-parametric variables were compared using the independent t-test and the Mann-Whitney U test, respectively. The paired t-test was used to compare findings before and after surgery. A p-value < 0.05 was considered statistically significant.

3. Results

All patients were divided into non-dacryoendoscopy and dacryoendoscopy groups (groups A and B, respectively) during STI. All patients underwent evaluation of tear secretion, usually before the age of 36 months. The clinical characteristics and demographic data of all subjects are listed in Table 1. The overall success rate was 91.8%, but the rate was significantly higher in group B (97.0%) than in group A (88.5%) (p = 0.038). The mean age of groups A and B was 32.7 ± 28.9 and 39.8 ± 30.4 months, respectively (p = 0.064). The mean epiphora duration was 25.5 ± 24.0 and 25.7 ± 27.7 months in groups A and B, respectively (p = 0.124). Previous lacrimal sac massage was more common in group A than group B (p = 0.032); neither the previous probing nor the STI rate (both p = 0.124), nor the tube insertion duration (p = 0.209), differed between the groups. The follow-up period was 8.1 ± 2.8 months in group A and 8.1 ± 3.0 months in group B (p = 0.956).

Dacryoendoscopy revealed all simple Hasner membrane blockages (defined above) (Figure 1a). During nasal endoscopy, the membrane was readily perforated without resistance or bleeding (Figure 1b). In terms of complicated blockages (defined above), a sickle knife was used during endoscopy to remove thick, dense fibrotic membranes (Figure 1c,d). When stenosis was present, the inferior meatus was narrower than the dacryoendoscope (Figure 1e). However, when the scope was moved, the Hasner valve was perforated as easily as the thin membrane of the simple type (Figure 1f). Sometimes, dacryoendoscopy revealed dacryoliths in the lacrimal sac (Figure 1g); these were fragmented under dacryoendoscopic guidance, the fragments were flushed out with saline, and success was confirmed by nasal endoscopy (Figure 1h).

Table 1. Clinical characteristics and demography in the patients according to the use of dacryoendoscopy.

	Group A (without Dacryoendoscopy)			Group B (with Dacryoendoscopy)			p
	≤36 Months	>36 Months	Total	≤36 Months	>36 Months	Total	
Age (month)	21.4 ± 7.3	63.5 ± 41.5	32.7 ± 28.9	22.6 ± 8.5	79.4 ± 24.9	39.8 ± 30.4	0.064
Patient-level characteristics	N = 30	N = 11	N = 41	N = 19	N = 9	N = 28	
Sex (male:female)	18:12	2:9	20:21	10:9	6:3	16:12	0.349
Epiphora duration (months)	18.1 ± 8.5	45.6 ± 38.1	25.5 ± 24.0	21.5 ± 9.0	47.1 ± 38.3	25.7 ± 27.7	0.124
Eye-level characteristics	N = 38	N = 14	N = 52	N = 23	N = 10	N = 33	
Laterality							
Unilateral (%)	24 (63.2)	8 (57.1)	32 (61.5)	17 (73.9)	8 (80.0)	25 (75.8)	0.174
Bilateral (%)	14 (36.8)	6 (42.9)	20 (38.5)	6 (26.1)	2 (20.0)	8 (24.2)	
Previous massage							
Yes (%)	5 (13.2)	0 (0.0)	5 (9.6)	6 (26.1)	3 (30.0)	9 (27.3)	0.032 *
No (%)	33 (86.8)	14 (100.0)	47 (90.4)	17 (73.9)	7 (70.0)	24 (72.7)	
Previous probing or STI							
Yes (%)	1 (2.6)	5 (35.7)	6 (11.5)	5 (21.7)	3 (30.0)	8 (24.2)	0.124
No (%)	37 (97.4)	9 (64.3)	46 (88.5)	18 (78.3)	7 (70.0)	25 (75.8)	
Duration of tube insertion (months)	5.3 ± 0.9	5.1 ± 1.9	5.2 ± 1.7	4.7 ± 3.4	4.2 ± 1.2	4.5 ± 2.8	0.209
Follow-up period (months)	8.1 ± 2.8	8.0 ± 2.9	8.1 ± 2.8	7.5 ± 2.9	8.1 ± 2.7	7.7 ± 2.6	0.426
Success rate (%)	32 (84.2)	14 (100.0)	46 (88.5)	23 (100.0)	9 (90.0)	32 (97.0)	0.038 *

STI: silicone tube intubation, *: $p < 0.05$.

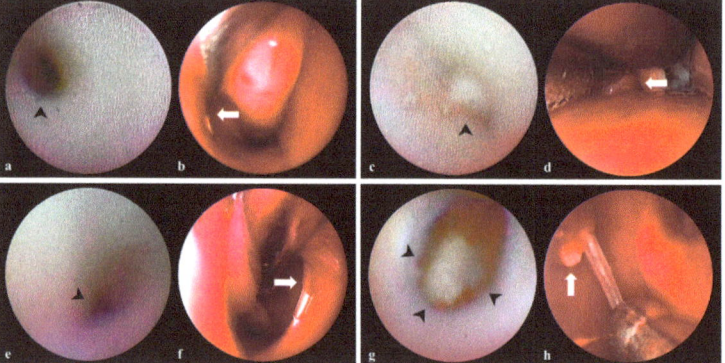

Figure 1. Classification of dacryoendoscopic findings (**a,c,e,g**) with nasoendoscopic findings (**b,d,f,h**) at the distal end of the nasolacrimal duct in patients with congenital nasolacrimal duct obstruction. Simple type presented, the normal lacrimal duct (arrowhead) in the right eye (**a**) and easily perforated at Hasner's valve (arrow) (**b**). Complicated type demonstrated dense fibrosis in the left lacrimal duct (arrowhead) (**c**) and thick fibrous membrane was removed using a sickle knife (arrow) (**d**). Stenosis type was noted before the left inferior meatus (arrowhead) (**e**) and thin membrane was readily perforated at Hasner's valve (arrow) (**f**). Dacryolith was noted at the right lacrimal sac (arrowhead) (**g**) and fragments of dacryolith were removed (arrow) (**h**).

The morphology of the distal end of the lacrimal duct was simple in twenty-four eyes (72.7%) and complicated in seven eyes (21.2%), including four (12.1%) with fibrosis and three (9.1%) with stenosis. Dacryoliths were encountered in two eyes (6.1%) (Figure 2a). Complicated LDS obstructions were found in the canaliculus (43%), lacrimal sac (43%), and lacrimal punctum (14%) (Figure 2b).

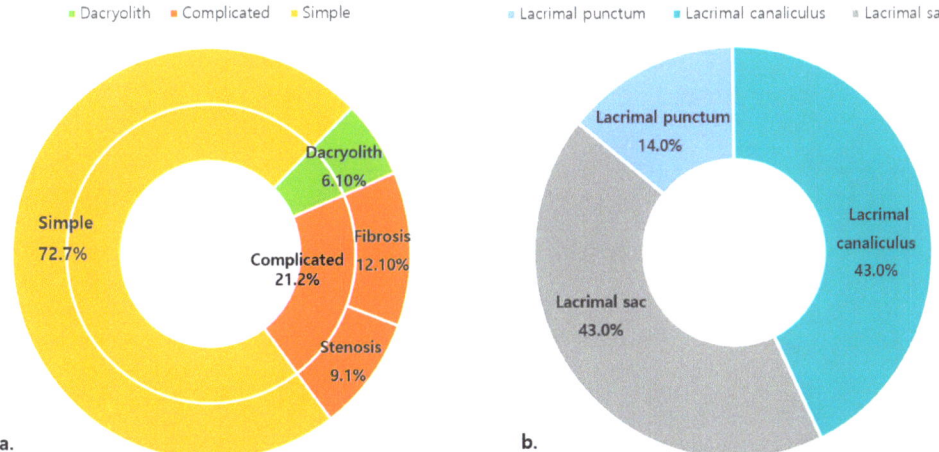

Figure 2. Distribution of the patients with congenital nasolacrimal duct obstruction. (**a**) Type of obstruction at the end of nasolacrimal duct by dacryoendoscopy (n = 33). (**b**) Level of obstruction in the lacrimal drainage system in the complicated type (n = 7).

The LDS obstructions were classified by the dacryoendoscopic findings. All LDS patterns were associated with either simple or complicated Hasner's valve obstructions. Sixteen eyes (48.5%) with stenosis exhibited simple obstructions. Among eleven eyes (33.3%) with mucus, eight and three had simple and complicated Hasner's valve features, respectively. Four eyes (12.1%) with membranes and two (6.1%) with dacryoliths exhibited complicated Hasner's valve features (Figure 3a). The LDS obstructive levels were as follows: canaliculus, 42.4%; sac, 39.4%; and nasolacrimal duct, 21.2%. The LDS obstructions were structural (n = 18) or secretory (n = 15) (Figure 3b).

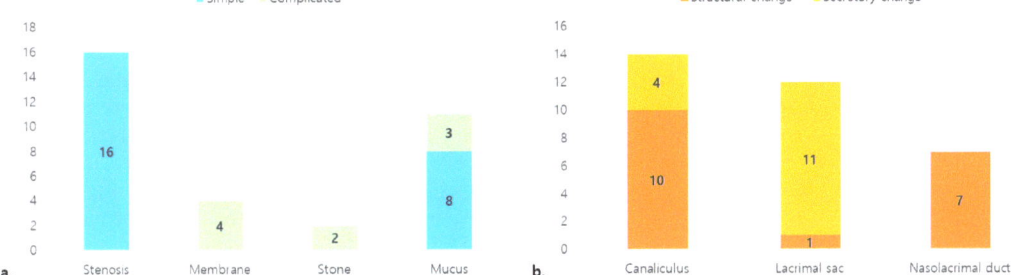

Figure 3. Correlation of dacryoendoscopic findings of the lacrimal drainage system and the type of congenital nasolacrimal duct obstruction. (**a**) Pattern of obstruction in the lacrimal drainage system according to the type of obstruction at the distal end of the nasolacrimal duct. (**b**) Level of obstruction in the lacrimal drainage system according to the pattern of obstruction.

LDS dacryoendoscopy revealed Hasner valve membranes in seven eyes (21.2%). All subjects were younger than 36 months and exhibited LDS structural obstructions. Twenty-six eyes (78.8%) without Hasner valve membranes exhibited both secretory and structural LDS obstructions regardless of age (Table 2). The correlation between the presence of a Hasner valve membrane and the LDS obstruction pattern on dacryoendoscopy was significant ($p = 0.049$). During the postoperative follow-up period, there were no complications related to STI, such as nasal hematoma, punctum erosion, and granuloma formation.

Table 2. Dacryoendoscopic findings in the lacrimal drainage system associated with the membrane at the Hasner's valve.

	Present (n = 7)				Absent (n = 26)				Total (n = 33)	p
	≤36 Months	>36 Months	Total	p	≤36 Months	>36 Months	Total	p		
Secretory change	0 (0.0)	0 (0.0)	0 (0.0)	NC	8 (50.0)	5 (50.0)	13 (50.0)	1.000	13 (37.1)	
Structural change	7 (100.0)	0 (0.0)	7 (100.0)		8 (50.0)	5 (50.0)	13 (50.0)		20 (62.9)	
Total	7 (100.0)	0 (0.0)	7 (100.0)		16 (61.5)	10 (38.5)	26 (100.0)		33 (100.0)	0.049 *

4. Discussion

We compared CNDO patients who underwent STI without and with dacryoendoscopy. The success rate was significantly higher in the latter group, at 97.0%, even though the rate of prior lacrimal sac massage was higher. The previous probing rate tended to be higher in the group that underwent dacryoendoscopy. Probing can be associated with false passage formation, LDS injury, and bleeding [17]. Thus, dacryoendoscopy would be expected to be more difficult in such patients. However, the better results of our dacryoendoscopy group can be explained by the real-time views of the pathologies; it was possible to visualize the entire LDS, including Hasner valve membranes. We also used nasal endoscopy to directly visualize the inferior nasal meatus; this assisted the localization of anatomical defects. This approach reduces the risks associated with blind intubation, including hemorrhage, nasal mucosal trauma, and iatrogenic false passage creation at the inferior opening of the nasolacrimal duct [18]. However, there was one failure in the dacryoendoscopic group. The symptoms of a 4-year-old boy improved only after STI, but epiphora recurred after extubation. The irrigation test revealed a good flow, indicating a satisfactory functional condition.

Our patients ranged in age from 11 to 123 months (average age = 45.0 ± 34.2 months) and were thus slightly older than the patients in other studies. Gupta et al. performed dacryoendoscopy on patients aged 9–36 months; the success rate was 100% [13]. Heichel et al. performed dacryoendoscopy on patients aged 1–12 months; the success rate was 94.4% [19]. Matsumura et al. reported an overall success rate of 100% in children aged 1–5 years [14]. As in previous studies, our success rate with patients aged < 36 months was 100%. Araz et al. [20] reported a significant difference in the minimum transverse diameter (in the sagittal plane) of the bony nasolacrimal canal duct between children < 2 and >3 years of age. By 36 months of age, the lacrimal system is fully developed, and LDS pathologies become more complex, which is associated with more secretions and mucus. Also, nasal inflammation caused by allergic rhinitis may affect the disease course, and tearing may be attributable to blepharitis, an epibleparon, keratitis, or foreign bodies [3].

Notably, our dacryoendoscopic CNDO findings were diverse, particularly in terms of the morphology of the distal end of the Hasner valve membrane, as previously reported [21]. Adult NDO levels and patterns vary to a greater extent than those of children because the causes of NDO are more diverse in adults. For example, the lacrimal duct is the most common site of adult obstruction, but this is not the case in children who have CNDO. However, even in children, it is essential to evaluate both the LDS and the Hasner valve when exploring NDO via both dacryoendoscopy and nasal endoscopy; the conventional blind intubation technique is no longer considered appropriate.

In terms of the pathological LDS changes, of the twenty eyes in this study exhibiting stenosis and membranes, sixteen were simple and four were complicated. Notably, all patients with stenosis were in the simple group, and all patients with membranes were in the complicated group. Of thirteen eyes with secretory patterns (mucus and stones), eight were simple and five were complicated. Thus, when the LDS is narrow or stenotic, as revealed by dacryoendoscopy, the Hasner valve membrane can easily be perforated provided LDS damage is carefully avoided. However, if the LDS exhibits a secretory pathology, the Hasner valve membrane may be complicated to deal with. It is essential to treat a fibrotic or stenotic membrane at the end of the NLD opening to ensure a favorable outcome.

This study had several limitations. It was a retrospective single-institution study with a small sample size, and further studies are needed. Also, all of the children were Korean; generalization of our findings to other populations should be carried out with caution. Finally, it was difficult to compare the CNDO types between the two groups because data on the Hasner valve and LDS obstructions in the conventional group were lacking. Future research will be needed to elucidate the pathological mechanisms causing changes within the LDS in CNDO.

In conclusion, STI combined with transcanalicular dacryoplasty was more successful than the conventional technique (without dacryoendoscopy). The CNDO etiopathologies identified by dacryoendoscopy were diverse, not only at the Hasner valve membrane but also throughout the LDS. Dacryoendoscopy-based direct visualization and recanalization effectively improve the STI outcomes of CNDO patients, particularly those younger than 36 months.

Author Contributions: Study Concept and Design (D.K. and H.L.); Collection and Management of Data (D.K.); Analysis and Interpretation of Data (D.K. and H.L.); Statistical Analysis (D.K.); Writing and Review of the Manuscript (D.K. and H.L.). All authors have read and agreed to the published version of the manuscript.

Funding: This research received no external funding.

Institutional Review Board Statement: The study and the data collection protocol were approved by the Institutional Review Board of CHA Bundang Medical Center, Seongnam, South Korea (approval no. 2023-09-035, approval date 31 October 2023). The study adhered to the tenets of the Declaration of Helsinki.

Informed Consent Statement: Informed consent was obtained from all parents or guardians prior to patient enrolment.

Data Availability Statement: The datasets analyzed during the current study are available from the corresponding author on reasonable requests.

Conflicts of Interest: The authors declare no conflict of interest.

References

1. Young, J.D.; MacEwen, C.J. Managing congenital lacrimal obstruction in general practice. *BMJ* **1997**, *315*, 293–296. [CrossRef] [PubMed]
2. Robb, R.M. Congenital nasolacrimal duct obstruction. *Ophthalmol. Clin. N. Am.* **2001**, *14*, 443–446. [CrossRef] [PubMed]
3. Schnall, B.M. Pediatric nasolacrimal duct obstruction. *Curr. Opin. Ophthalmol.* **2013**, *24*, 421–424. [CrossRef] [PubMed]
4. Aldahash, F.D.; Al-Mubarak, M.F.; Alenizi, S.H.; Al-Faky, Y.H. Risk factors for developing congenital nasolacrimal duct obstruction. *Saudi J. Ophthalmol.* **2014**, *28*, 58–60. [CrossRef] [PubMed]
5. Pediatric Eye Disease Investigator, G. Resolution of congenital nasolacrimal duct obstruction with nonsurgical management. *Arch. Ophthalmol.* **2012**, *130*, 730–734. [CrossRef] [PubMed]
6. Sathiamoorthi, S.; Frank, R.D.; Mohney, B.G. Spontaneous Resolution and Timing of Intervention in Congenital Nasolacrimal Duct Obstruction. *JAMA Ophthalmol.* **2018**, *136*, 1281–1286. [CrossRef]
7. Bansal, O.; Bothra, N.; Sharma, A.; Ali, M.J. Congenital nasolacrimal duct obstruction update study (CUP study): Paper II—Profile and outcomes of complex CNLDO and masquerades. *Int. J. Pediatr. Otorhinolaryngol.* **2020**, *139*, 110407. [CrossRef]
8. Vagge, A.; Ferro Desideri, L.; Nucci, P.; Serafino, M.; Giannaccare, G.; Lembo, A.; Traverso, C.E. Congenital Nasolacrimal Duct Obstruction (CNLDO): A Review. *Diseases* **2018**, *6*, 96. [CrossRef]
9. MacEwen, C.J.; Young, J.D. Epiphora during the first year of life. *Eye* **1997**, *5 Pt 5*, 596–600. [CrossRef]
10. Heichel, J.; Bredehorn-Mayr, T.; Struck, H.G. Congenital nasolacrimal duct obstruction from an ophthalmologist's point of view: Causes, diagnosis and staged therapeutic concept. *HNO* **2016**, *64*, 367–375. [CrossRef]
11. Swierczynska, M.; Tobiczyk, E.; Rodak, P.; Barchanowska, D.; Filipek, E. Success rates of probing for congenital nasolacrimal duct obstruction at various ages. *BMC Ophthalmol.* **2020**, *20*, 403. [CrossRef] [PubMed]
12. Gardiner, J.A.; Forte, V.; Pashby, R.C.; Levin, A.V. The role of nasal endoscopy in repeat pediatric nasolacrimal duct probings. *J. AAPOS* **2001**, *5*, 148–152. [CrossRef] [PubMed]

13. Gupta, N.; Singla, P.; Kumar, S.; Ganesh, S.; Dhawan, N.; Sobti, P.; Aggarwal, S. Role of dacryoendoscopy in refractory cases of congenital nasolacrimal duct obstruction. *Orbit* **2020**, *39*, 183–189. [CrossRef] [PubMed]
14. Matsumura, N.; Suzuki, T.; Goto, S.; Fujita, T.; Yamane, S.; Maruyama-Inoue, M.; Kadonosono, K. Transcanalicular endoscopic primary dacryoplasty for congenital nasolacrimal duct obstruction. *Eye* **2019**, *33*, 1008–1013. [CrossRef] [PubMed]
15. Li, Y.; Wei, M.; Liu, X.; Zhang, L.; Song, X.; Xiao, C. Dacryoendoscopy-assisted incision of Hasner's valve under nasoendoscopy for membranous congenital nasolacrimal duct obstruction after probing failure: A retrospective study. *BMC Ophthalmol.* **2021**, *21*, 182. [CrossRef] [PubMed]
16. Kim, D.A.; Lew, H. Dacryoendoscopic Findings in the Failed Silicone Tube Intubations without Dacryoendoscopy. *Korean J. Ophthalmol.* **2022**, *36*, 486–492. [CrossRef]
17. Petris, C.; Liu, D. Probing for congenital nasolacrimal duct obstruction. *Cochrane Database Syst. Rev.* **2017**, *7*, CD011109. [CrossRef]
18. Arici, C.; Oto, B.B. Nasal endospy-guided primary nasolacrimal duct intubation for congenital nasolacrimal duct obstruction in children older than 4 years. *Int. Ophthalmol.* **2023**, *43*, 1005–1011. [CrossRef]
19. Heichel, J.; Struck, H.G.; Fiorentzis, M.; Hammer, T.; Bredehorn-Mayr, T. A Case Series of Dacryoendoscopy in Childhood: A Diagnostic and Therapeutic Alternative for Complex Congenital Nasolacrimal Duct Obstruction Even in the First Year of Life. *Adv. Ther.* **2017**, *34*, 1221–1232. [CrossRef]
20. Ela, A.S.; Cigdem, K.E.; Karagoz, Y.; Yigit, O.; Longur, E.S. Morphometric Measurements of Bony Nasolacrimal Canal in Children. *J. Craniofac. Surg.* **2018**, *29*, e282–e287. [CrossRef]
21. Lee, S.M.; Lew, H. Transcanalicular endoscopic dacryoplasty in patients with primary acquired nasolacrimal duct obstruction. *Graefes. Arch. Clin. Exp. Ophthalmol.* **2021**, *259*, 173–180. [CrossRef] [PubMed]

Disclaimer/Publisher's Note: The statements, opinions and data contained in all publications are solely those of the individual author(s) and contributor(s) and not of MDPI and/or the editor(s). MDPI and/or the editor(s) disclaim responsibility for any injury to people or property resulting from any ideas, methods, instructions or products referred to in the content.

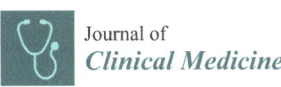

Article

Assessment of Office-Based Probing with Dacryoendoscopy for Treatment of Congenital Nasolacrimal Duct Obstruction: A Retrospective Study

Yoshiki Ueta *, Yuji Watanabe, Ryoma Kamada and Nobuya Tanaka

Department of Ophthalmology, Shinseikai Toyama Hospital, 89-10 Shimowaka, Imizu 939-0243, Toyama, Japan
* Correspondence: uetayoshiki@gmail.com; Tel.: +81-766-52-2156

Abstract: We aimed to evaluate the safety and efficacy of office-based probing with dacryoendoscopy under local anesthesia for congenital nasolacrimal duct obstruction (CNLDO). This single-institution study retrospectively reviewed data on 72 eyes of 64 consecutive children (38 boys, 43 eyes; 26 girls, 29 eyes), aged between 6 and 17 (mean age: 10.0 ± 2.7) months with suspected CNLDO, from July 2016 to February 2022. These patients underwent probing with dacryoendoscopy under local anesthesia. CNLDO was diagnosed clinically based on the presence of epiphora and sticky eyes due to mucous discharge commencing within the first 3 months of life, increased tear meniscus height, and fluorescein dye disappearance test results. A total of 63 of the 72 eyes had narrowly defined CNLDO, and 9 eyes had other types of obstructions. The intervention success rate was 100% (63/63 eyes) for patients with typical CNLDO and 97.2% (70/72 eyes) for the entire study cohort. Moreover, CNLDO was classified into five types based on the features of the distal end of the nasolacrimal duct. Probing with dacryoendoscopy is safe and yields a high success rate in pediatric patients with CNLDO. This is the first study to assess the safety and efficacy of probing with dacryoendoscopy under local anesthesia in pediatric patients with CNLDO.

Keywords: congenital nasolacrimal duct obstruction; dacryoendoscopy; epiphora; local anesthesia; office probing

1. Introduction

Congenital nasolacrimal duct obstruction (CNLDO) is characterized by congenital membranous blockage of the distal end of the nasolacrimal duct [1]. The symptoms of CNLDO include epiphora or mucoid discharge from the eye within the first three months of life. Different variants of complex CNLDO exist, such as lacrimal punctum obstruction, agenesis of the lacrimal punctum, and bony obstruction. The incidence of CNLDO and lacrimal drainage dysfunction in infancy reportedly ranges from 6 to 20% [2–4].

Blind probing is the first choice of surgical treatment for CNLDO; however, the optimal timing of probing is being debated worldwide [5,6]. Spontaneous resolution of CNLDO by 12 months of age has been reported to occur in 82–96% of patients [2,7]. Some experts suggest that conservative treatment with eye drops and a lacrimal sac massage be recommended for a specific waiting period to allow spontaneous resolution, and upon failing, surgical treatment should be recommended under general anesthesia. However, set-up for general anesthesia is not normally available in most of the facilities, particularly for infants, and if available, it is labor-intensive for parents, doctors, and hospital personnel. Therefore, blind probing under local anesthesia can be considered in children aged <1 year in facilities where treatment under general anesthesia is not feasible. The CNLDO guidelines established in 2022 in Japan also recommend probing under local anesthesia for children 6–9 months of age [8].

Probing is a blind procedure, and canalicular stenosis has been shown to develop in pediatric patients after unsuccessful initial probings [9]. In recent years, several studies

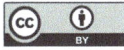

have evaluated dacryoendoscopy-guided probing for CNLDO [10–17], most of which were performed under general anesthesia. Since dacryoendoscopy allows for direct visualization of the lacrimal passage, this technique may facilitate safer and more reliable probing if performed under local anesthesia.

To the best of our knowledge, no previous study has examined the outcomes of probing with dacryoendoscopy, under local anesthesia in patients with CNLDO. Therefore, this is the first study that aimed to assess the safety and efficacy of this technique performed with local anesthesia in pediatric patients with CNLDO.

2. Materials and Methods

2.1. Ethics

This study was conducted in accordance with the tenets of the Declaration of Helsinki and approved by the Institutional Ethical Review Board of Shinseikai Toyama Hospital (approval number: 220223-1). We used an opt-out consent process by using the full written information about this research. Participants were included in the research unless their parents expressed their decision that they be excluded. The written full information was approved, and the requirement for obtaining informed consent was waived by the Institutional Review Board of Shinseikai Toyama Hospital.

2.2. Patients

We retrospectively reviewed the medical records of 72 eyes of 64 consecutive children (38 boys, 43 eyes; 26 girls, 29 eyes) aged between 6 and 17 (mean age: 10.0 ± 2.7) months with suspected CNLDO. These patients underwent probing with dacryoendoscopy under local anesthesia at our department between July 2016 and February 2022.

The clinical diagnosis of CNLDO was based on the presence of epiphora and sticky eye due to mucous discharge commencing within the first 3 months of life, increased tear meniscus height, and fluorescein dye disappearance test (FDDT) results. Additionally, the exclusion of a history of trichiasis, congenital glaucoma, keratitis, uveitis, and epidemic keratoconjunctivitis also assisted in establishing the clinical diagnosis of CNLDO. FDDT was performed as per the routine protocol [18]. Briefly, a drop of the fluorescein dye was instilled into the palpebral conjunctiva, and if the fluorescence persisted in the tear meniscus beyond 5 min, lacrimal drainage dysfunction was diagnosed. CNLDO might be ruled out if the fluorescent dye reached the nasal secretion due to the patency of the lacrimal duct. We did not perform lacrimal irrigation to diagnose CNLDO since it is an invasive procedure and uncomfortable for infants and children.

The parents of the children were instructed to perform lacrimal sac massage until 6 months of age, and we explained that they could request general anesthesia for their child if spontaneous resolution was not achieved until the age of 1 year or early probing under topical anesthesia. Probing was performed for patients for whom early intervention was requested. We limited patient enrollment to infants and young children who were not yet able to walk unaided.

2.3. Surgical Instruments

Dacryoendoscopy was performed using the MT-3000 device (FiberTech Co., Ltd., Tokyo, Japan) (Figure 1). The dacryoendoscope has a curved, rigid probe that contains a 3000-pixel fiberoptic bundle, illumination fibers, and irrigation channel. The probe length is 50 mm. The outer diameters of the root and tip measure 1.0 and 0.7 mm, respectively, with an angulation of 27° 10 mm from the tip. The MT-3000 possesses a tapered tip and yields images of low quality.

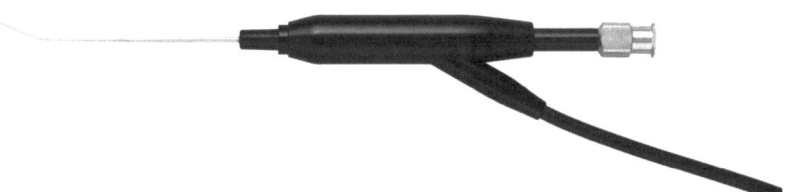

Figure 1. The MT-3000 dacryoendoscope (FiberTech Co., Tokyo, Japan) used in this study. This device has a tapered tip and acquires low-quality images (3000 pixels). The probe length is 50 mm, the outer diameter of the root is 1.0 mm, and the outer diameter of the tip is 0.7 mm, with an angulation of 27° 10 mm from the tip.

2.4. Surgical Procedure and Techniques

The surgical procedure employed in this study was as follows. A surgeon (Y.U.) skilled in dacryoendoscopic surgery performed the procedure, wherein ophthalmic anesthesia was induced via instillation of oxyprocaine and 4% lidocaine drops. Two caregivers restrained the patient with a retardation band. If the restraint was inadequate, the surgery was aborted. Insertion was achieved via the upper lacrimal punctum. The lower lacrimal punctum was used as the point of access in difficult cases. The lacrimal punctum was dilated using a punctal dilator, while the lacrimal sac was washed to eliminate as much pus as possible. The dacryoendoscope was inserted through the lacrimal punctum, and saline was injected to dilate the lacrimal canal while advancing the endoscope. Once the dacryoendoscope reached the lacrimal sac, the endoscope was held upright and advanced along the nasolacrimal duct to the distal end. The pus was then washed out to confirm the site of obstruction, followed by a puncture. If the obstruction site was difficult to confirm due to pus, a low-quality image, or body movement, semi-blind probing was attempted. Perforation was confirmed by assessing the nasal mucosa with the dacryoendoscope and by passing the saline solution. Antibiotic eye drops were administered for 3 days postoperatively. The children were followed up after 2 weeks to assess the patency of the lacrimal passage. Treatment success was defined as the disappearance of symptoms and a negative FDDT.

We have uploaded two videos of the procedure as supplementary material. Video S1 shows the dacryoendoscopic view of the patient with CNLDO in the left eye. The distal end of the nasolacrimal duct and the obstruction site are medial (Type 2). Video S2 shows the viewing of the dacryoendoscopic probing. The punctum is dilated and a dacryoendoscope is inserted, following which the obstruction site is perforated. It takes about 1–3 min from dilating the punctum to perforating and removing the dacryoendoscope. The Power Direct 365 program was used to create the videos.

2.5. Outcomes

The primary outcome was the rate of treatment success, defined as the disappearance of symptoms (epiphora and eye discharge) and a negative FDDT at 2 weeks post-surgery. The binomial proportion confidence intervals on the success rate were calculated for the 95% confidence interval (CI) using the Agresti–Coull method. The secondary outcomes included complications and endoscopic findings of the distal end of the nasolacrimal duct.

3. Results

The principal results of the study are presented in Table 1. A total of 63 of the 72 eyes had typical CNLDO (the term "typical" refers to congenital blockage of the distal end of the nasolacrimal duct, specifically the Hasner valve), and the remaining 9 eyes had other types of obstructions, including upper and lower lacrimal punctum obstruction (incomplete punctal canalization (IPC); $n = 4$). One of the four cases had IPC alone, two had combined distal end of the nasolacrimal duct obstruction, and one had combined inferior lacrimal canaliculus obstruction. The other five had common canaliculus obstruction ($n = 1$), lower nasolacrimal duct obstruction ($n = 3$), and lower nasolacrimal duct and inferior lacrimal canaliculus obstruction ($n = 1$).

Table 1. Comparative results of the obstruction site, sample size, and success rate.

Obstruction Site	n	Success Rate
Distal end of the nasolacrimal duct alone (typical CNLDO)	63	100% (63/63)
Upper and lower lacrimal punctum (IPC)		
IPC alone	1	100% (1/1)
Distal end of the nasolacrimal duct	2	100% (2/2)
Inferior lacrimal canaliculus	1	0% (0/1)
Common canaliculus	1	0% (0/1)
Lower nasolacrimal duct	3	100% (3/3)
Inferior lacrimal canaliculus and lower nasolacrimal duct	1	100% (1/1)
Total	72	97.2% (70/72)

CNLDO, congenital nasolacrimal duct obstruction; IPC, incomplete punctal canalization.

The success rate of probing using dacryoendoscopy for typical CNLDO was 100% (63/63 eyes). Punctum obstruction was not successfully opened in one eye with upper and lower IPC and inferior lacrimal canaliculus obstruction. However, the duct was opened, and re-obstruction was observed in one case (common canaliculus obstruction) at the 2-week follow-up visit. Resolution was achieved in all other cases of CNLDO. The success rate of intervention in the entire study cohort was 97.2% (70/72 eyes). The binomial proportion confidence intervals on the success rate are 89.8–99.8% for the 95% CI (using the Agresti–Coull method). Seven eyes of six patients had undergone prior initial probing at other hospitals, all of which showed complete resolution. Restraint was performed safely on all children up to 17 months of age. There were no cases with complications such as damage to the punctum and canaliculus, hyperemia, infections, or false passage.

The obstruction site could not be observed on the endoscopic image in 31 (49%) eyes of the 63 cases of typical CNLDO due to the following reasons: first, the obstruction was punctured before visualization of the site of obstruction (semi-blind); second, the site of obstruction was difficult to visualize due to the presence of pus or body movement; and third, the resolution of the dacryoendoscope was poor. The occlusion site could be visualized in the remaining 32 cases. Thirty and two cases of simple membranous and stenosis-type obstructions, respectively, were observed. The eyes were classified into five groups based on the findings of the nasolacrimal duct distal end obstruction sites (Figure 2). Type 1 included eyes with no dilation near the distal end of the nasolacrimal duct and obstruction in the center ($n = 2$). Type 2 comprised eyes with no dilation near the distal end of the nasolacrimal duct, and the obstruction site was medial ($n = 12$). Type 3 included eyes in which the distal end of the nasolacrimal duct was bent such that the obstructed site could not be observed from the front (irrespective of the presence or absence of dilation) ($n = 5$). Type 4 was characterized by dilation near the distal end of the nasolacrimal duct, and the obstruction site was medial ($n = 7$). Type 5 was characterized by dilation near the distal end of the nasolacrimal duct, and the obstruction site was in front of the nasal end (probably due to dilation near the distal end of the nasolacrimal duct; $n = 6$).

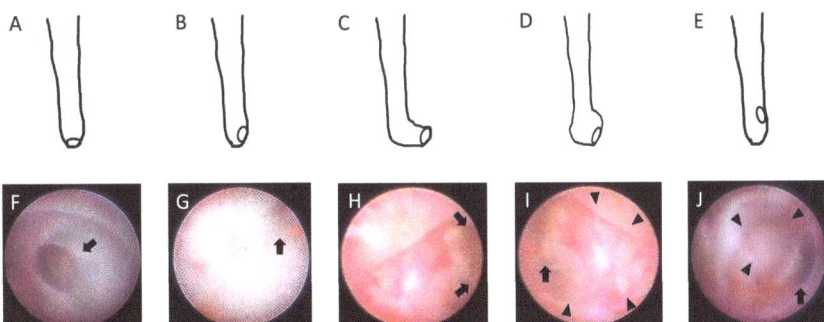

Figure 2. Classification of the distal end of the nasolacrimal duct by shape (illustrations and photographs). (**A,F**): Type 1, absence of dilation near the distal end of the nasolacrimal duct, and the obstructed valve of Hasner is located at the center (arrow). (**B,G**): Type 2, absence of dilation near the distal end of the nasolacrimal duct, and the obstructed valve of Hasner is medial (arrow). (**C,H**): Type 3, the distal end of the nasolacrimal duct is bent such that the obstructed site (beyond the arrow) cannot be seen from the front (irrespective of the presence or absence of dilation). (**D,I**): Type 4, presence of dilation near the distal end of the nasolacrimal duct (arrowheads), and the obstructed valve of Hasner is medial (arrow). (**E,J**): Type 5, presence of dilation near the distal end of the nasolacrimal duct (arrowheads), and the obstructed valve of Hasner is located in front of the nasal end (arrow). The small circles in (**A–E**) indicate the location of the obstruction, specifically the Hasner valve, with the nasal cavity located behind it. The CLIP STUDIO graphics program was used to create the illustration.

4. Discussion

Herein, we report the first study to assess the safety and success rates of probing with dacryoendoscopy under local anesthesia in pediatric patients with CNLDO. The success rate of intervention in the entire patient population was 97.2% (70/72 eyes) and 100% in the eyes with typical CNLDO (63/63 eyes). The binomial proportion confidence intervals on the success rate are 89.8–99.8% for the 95% CI.

Fujimoto et al. [13] reported a 98.1% success rate with dacryoendoscopic probing in 54 CNLDO cases, including refractory disease. Matsumura et al. [14] also reported a 100% success rate for dacryoendoscopic probing under general anesthesia in 56 cases. The success rate of blind probing is 75–92% [5,19–24], and if limited to office probing, the success rate is 75–88.6% [21–24]. In comparison, dacryoendoscopic probing may have a relatively higher success rate.

The site of obstruction could be visualized in 32 cases, and based on this, CNLDO was classified into five types. It is not difficult to perforate the obstruction in types 1 and 2, even with blind probing. However, puncturing is difficult with normal blind probing in types 3 to 5 because the blockage is not located at the distal end of the duct. It may even be impossible to penetrate the blockage in types 3 and 5 without using dacryoendoscopy. Matsumura et al. [14] reported that the precise location of the blockage in the simple type was approximately 0.5–1.0 mm proximal to the end of the duct. In addition, the duct sometimes ends with a "pocket" in the nasal mucosa of the lateral wall of the nasal cavity. This particular anatomical configuration could be considered as a factor contributing to the failure of probing using the blind technique. It is thought that the failure rate of blind probing may be high in types 3, 4, and 5; the use of dacryoendoscopy can prevent misdirected probing, thus improving the success rate. Furthermore, dilation near the distal end of the nasolacrimal duct was another feature that could be visualized using dacryoendoscopy. It is unclear whether this dilation was an original feature or an abnormal manifestation of chronic inflammation. Given that distal end dilation is frequently absent in adult dacryoendoscopic observations, this dilation may be a consequence of chronic inflammation that tends to revert to its characteristic shape with the subsidence of the inflammation. The greater the severity of the dilation, the greater the degree of displacement of the obstruction site. It has been reported that the success rate of interventions decreases with increasing age [20]. This may be attributed to changes in the shape of the distal end of the nasolacrimal duct due to chronic inflammation.

We used the MT-3000 device (FiberTech Co., Ltd., Tokyo, Japan) as the dacryoendoscope, which had a curved, rigid probe containing a 3000-pixel fiberoptic bundle. The outer diameters of the root and tip measured 1.0 and 0.7 mm, respectively, with an angulation of 27°, 10 mm from the tip. The MT-3000 features a tapered tip but yields low-quality images. Conventional dacryoendoscopes typically employ a straight-type probe, but in Japan, a bent-type probe has been developed [8]. In terms of resolution rate, five studies [10,11,13–15] that used a curved dacryoendoscope have reported success rates that are fairly consistent across the studies (ranging from 92.3% to 100%). On the other hand, among the three studies [12,16,17] that utilized a straight dacryoendoscope, success rates varied from 53.8% to 94.4%. While there are no randomized control trials that investigate the impact of the shape of the handpiece of a dacryoendoscope on success rates, there is a tendency for the success rate to be higher when curved dacryoendoscopes are used. Anatomically, the lacrimal duct is curved, and curved dacryoendoscopes can visualize these lacrimal ducts more accurately. Hence, we believe that using a bent-type dacryoendoscope is preferable for endoscopic probing of the lacrimal duct. Additionally, the MT-3000 has a tapered tip and provides low-quality images. Better resolution is essential for effectively identifying obstruction sites. In some cases, in our study, the obstruction site was difficult to identify due to this low resolution. However, in children, the lacrimal punctums are smaller than in adults. Furthermore, when operating under local anesthesia, it is desirable to use a less invasive technique to keep the duration of the procedure as short as possible. Consequently, we prioritized ease of insertion and used a dacryoendoscope with a tapered 0.7 mm tip. When dacryoendoscopic probing is performed under general anesthesia, it is advisable to employ a dacryoendoscope with a higher resolution.

Compared with blind probing, dacryoendoscopic probing requires preparation for dacryoendoscopy, skill, and larger lacrimal punctum dilation and has no advantage for upper lacrimal system obstruction. In addition, it is not a substitute for dacryoendoscopic probing under general anesthesia because of the age limitation and the inability to insert a lacrimal tube. However, dacryoendoscopic probing under topical anesthesia is a short procedure that usually takes 2–3 min, from dilating the punctum to perforating and removing the dacryoendoscope, and nasolacrimal duct visualization can be achieved. The advantages of dacryoendoscopic probing over blind probing under local anesthesia include the ability to (1) reach the distal end of the nasolacrimal duct without creating a false pathway, (2) respond to the shape of the distal end of the nasolacrimal duct, and (3) find and treat obstructions in areas other than the distal end of the nasolacrimal duct (such as upper or lower nasolacrimal duct obstruction and dacryolith). Moreover, dacryoendoscopic probing under general anesthesia is limited due to a lack of appropriate facilities that can provide general anesthesia in children. Furthermore, general anesthesia is expensive and associated with complications. Therefore, office-based dacryoendoscopic probing under topical anesthesia may be an alternative to conventional blind probing and dacryoendoscopic probing under general anesthesia.

This study has several limitations. First, it incorporated a retrospective case series design, and there is no control group like blind probing. Second, patients were followed up for only 2 weeks after surgery. Subsequent re-occlusion might have occurred, which was not evaluated in this study. However, once the correct duct is opened, re-occlusion is unlikely to occur in patients with typical CNLDO [20,25]. Therefore, we believe that follow-up examinations 2 weeks postoperatively are sufficient if accurate puncturing is ensured during surgery. Third, our results may not be generalizable to all clinicians because the operation of the dacryoendoscopy requires suitable skills. Fourth, since families that select general anesthesia may have risk factors for failure in the clinic, the study's opt-out design may induce bias toward favorable results. Within the scope of these limitations, this study demonstrated the safety and high success rate of office probing with dacryoendoscopy. Therefore, this technique should be considered at facilities where general anesthesia is not available.

5. Conclusions

Probing with dacryoendoscopy has a high success rate and can be considered as a safe treatment modality for CNLDO. Although it is necessary to become proficient with the instruments and handling of the dacryoendoscopy, this technique may be recommended at facilities where general anesthesia is not available.

Supplementary Materials: The following supporting information can be downloaded at: https://www.mdpi.com/article/10.3390/jcm12227048/s1, Video S1: dacryoendoscopic view; Video S2: View of dacryoendoscopic probing.

Author Contributions: Y.U. treated the patients, collected the clinical data, and analyzed the findings. Y.W., R.K. and N.T. provided critical suggestions. All the authors agree to be accountable for all aspects of the work. All authors have read and agreed to the published version of the manuscript.

Funding: This research received no external funding.

Institutional Review Board Statement: This study was conducted in accordance with the tenets of the Declaration of Helsinki and approved by the Institutional Ethical Review Board of Shinseikai Toyama Hospital (approval number: 220223-1).

Informed Consent Statement: We used an opt-out consent process, and the requirement for obtaining informed consent was waived by the Institutional Review Board of Shinseikai Toyama Hospital.

Data Availability Statement: All data analyzed in this study are included in this article. Further inquiries can be directed to the corresponding author.

Acknowledgments: We would like to express our gratitude to the individuals who contributed to the refinement of this manuscript.

Conflicts of Interest: The authors declare no conflict of interest.

Abbreviations

CNLDO	congenital nasolacrimal duct obstruction
FDDT	fluorescein dye disappearance test
IPC	incomplete punctal canalization

References

1. Young, J.D.; MacEwen, C.J. Managing Congenital Lacrimal Obstruction in General Practice. *BMJ* **1997**, *315*, 293–296. [CrossRef]
2. MacEwen, C.J.; Young, J.D. Epiphora during the First Year of Life. *Eye* **1991**, *5*, 596–600. [CrossRef] [PubMed]
3. Noda, S.; Hayasaka, S.; Setogawa, T. Congenital Nasolacrimal Duct Obstruction in Japanese Infants: Its Incidence and Treatment with Massage. *J. Pediatr. Ophthalmol. Strabismus* **1991**, *28*, 20–22. [PubMed]
4. Kapadia, M.K.; Freitag, S.K.; Woog, J.J. Evaluation and Management of Congenital Nasolacrimal Duct Obstruction. *Otolaryngol. Clin. N. Am.* **2006**, *39*, 959–977. [CrossRef]
5. Pediatric Eye Disease Investigator Group. A Randomized Trial Comparing the Cost-Effectiveness of 2 Approaches for Treating Unilateral Nasolacrimal Duct Obstruction. *Arch. Ophthalmol.* **2012**, *130*, 1525–1533. [CrossRef] [PubMed]
6. Petris, C.; Liu, D. Probing for Congenital Nasolacrimal Duct Obstruction. *Cochrane Database Syst. Rev.* **2017**, *7*, CD011109. [CrossRef]
7. Kakizaki, H.; Takahashi, Y.; Kinoshita, S.; Shiraki, K.; Iwaki, M. The Rate of Symptomatic Improvement of Congenital Nasolacrimal Duct Obstruction in Japanese Infants Treated with Conservative Management during the 1st Year of Age. *Clin. Ophthalmol.* **2008**, *2*, 291–294. [CrossRef]
8. Pediatric Eye Disease Investigator Group. Guideline Committee for Congenital Nasolacrimal Duct Obstruction. A Guideline for Congenital Nasolacrimal Duct Obstruction in Japan. *Nippon Ganka Gakkai Zasshi* **2022**, *126*, 991–921.
9. Lyon, D.B.; Dortzbach, R.K.; Lemke, B.N.; Gonnering, R.S. Canalicular Stenosis Following Probing for Congenital Nasolacrimal Duct Obstruction. *Ophthalmic Surg.* **1991**, *22*, 228–232.
10. Sasaki, H.; Takano, T.; Murakami, A. Direct Endoscopic Probing for Congenital Lacrimal Duct Obstruction. *Clin. Exp. Ophthalmol.* **2013**, *41*, 729–734. [CrossRef]

11. Kato, K.; Matsunaga, K.; Takashima, Y.; Kondo, M. Probing of Congenital Nasolacrimal Duct Obstruction with Dacryoendoscope. *Clin. Ophthalmol.* **2014**, *8*, 977–980. [CrossRef] [PubMed]
12. Gupta, N.; Singla, P.; Kumar, S.; Ganesh, S.; Dhawan, N.; Sobti, P.; Aggarwal, S. Role of Dacryoendoscopy in Refractory Cases of Congenital Nasolacrimal Duct Obstruction. *Orbit* **2020**, *39*, 183–189. [CrossRef] [PubMed]
13. Fujimoto, M.; Ogino, K.; Matsuyama, H.; Miyazaki, C. Success Rates of Dacryoendoscopy-Guided Probing for Recalcitrant Congenital Nasolacrimal Duct Obstruction. *Jpn. J. Ophthalmol.* **2016**, *60*, 274–279. [CrossRef] [PubMed]
14. Matsumura, N.; Suzuki, T.; Goto, S.; Fujita, T.; Yamane, S.; Maruyama-Inoue, M.; Kadonosono, K. Transcanalicular Endoscopic Primary Dacryoplasty for Congenital Nasolacrimal Duct Obstruction. *Eye* **2019**, *33*, 1008–1013. [CrossRef]
15. Li, Y.; Wei, M.; Liu, X.; Zhang, L.; Song, X.; Xiao, C. Dacryoendoscopy-Assisted Incision of Hasner's Valve under Nasoendoscopy for Membranous Congenital Nasolacrimal Duct Obstruction after Probing Failure: A Retrospective Study. *BMC Ophthalmol.* **2021**, *21*, 182. [CrossRef]
16. Gupta, N.; Singla, P.; Ganesh, S. Usefulness of High Definition Sialoendoscope for Evaluation of Lacrimal Drainage System in Congenital Nasolacrimal Duct Obstruction. *Eur. J. Ophthalmol.* **2021**, *32*, 11206721211008047. [CrossRef]
17. Heichel, J.; Struck, H.G.; Fiorentzis, M.; Hammer, T.; Bredehorn-Mayr, T. A Case Series of Dacryoendoscopy in Childhood: A Diagnostic and Therapeutic Alternative for Complex Congenital Nasolacrimal Duct Obstruction Even in the First Year of Life. *Adv. Ther.* **2017**, *34*, 1221–1232. [CrossRef]
18. MacEwen, C.J.; Young, J.D. The Fluorescein Disappearance Test (FDT): An Evaluation of Its Use in Infants. *J. Pediatr. Ophthalmol. Strabismus* **1991**, *28*, 302–305. [CrossRef]
19. Al-Faky, Y.H.; Mousa, A.; Kalantan, H.; Al-Otaibi, A.; Alodan, H.; Alsuhaibani, A.H. A Prospective, Randomised Comparison of Probing versus Bicanalicular Silastic Intubation for Congenital Nasolacrimal Duct Obstruction. *Br. J. Ophthalmol.* **2015**, *99*, 246–250. [CrossRef]
20. Perveen, S.; Sufi, A.R.; Rashid, S.; Khan, A. Success Rate of Probing for Congenital Nasolacrimal Duct Obstruction at Various Ages. *J. Ophthalmic Vis. Res.* **2014**, *9*, 60–69.
21. Cha, D.S.; Lee, H.; Park, M.S.; Lee, J.M.; Baek, S.H. Clinical Outcomes of Initial and Repeated Nasolacrimal Duct Office-Based Probing for Congenital Nasolacrimal Duct Obstruction. *Korean J. Ophthalmol.* **2010**, *24*, 261–266. [CrossRef] [PubMed]
22. Miller, A.M.; Chandler, D.L.; Repka, M.X.; Hoover, D.L.; Lee, K.A.; Melia, M.; Rychwalski, P.J.; Silbert, D.I.; Pediatric Eye Disease Investigator Group; Beck, R.W.; et al. Office Probing for Treatment of Nasolacrimal Duct Obstruction in Infants. *J. AAPOS* **2014**, *18*, 26–30. [CrossRef] [PubMed]
23. Hung, C.H.; Chen, Y.C.; Lin, S.L.; Chen, W.L. Nasolacrimal Duct Probing Under Topical Anesthesia for Congenital Nasolacrimal Duct Obstruction in Taiwan. *Pediatr. Neonatol.* **2015**, *56*, 402–407. [CrossRef] [PubMed]
24. Lee, C.; Jeong, S.M.; Kim, G.J.; Joo, E.Y.; Song, M.H.; Sa, H.S. Efficacy and Safety of Inhalation Sedation During Office Probing for Congenital Nasolacrimal Duct Obstruction. *J. Clin. Med.* **2021**, *10*, 1800. [CrossRef]
25. Kashkouli, M.B.; Beigi, B.; Parvaresh, M.M.; Kassaee, A.; Tabatabaee, Z. Late and Very Late Initial Probing for Congenital Nasolacrimal Duct Obstruction: What Is the Cause of Failure? *Br. J. Ophthalmol.* **2003**, *87*, 1151–1153. [CrossRef]

Disclaimer/Publisher's Note: The statements, opinions and data contained in all publications are solely those of the individual author(s) and contributor(s) and not of MDPI and/or the editor(s). MDPI and/or the editor(s) disclaim responsibility for any injury to people or property resulting from any ideas, methods, instructions or products referred to in the content.

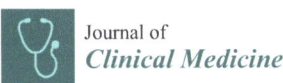

Article

Surgical Outcomes of Bilateral Inferior Rectus Muscle Recession for Restrictive Strabismus Secondary to Thyroid Eye Disease

Steffani Krista Someda [1], Naomi Umezawa [1,2], Aric Vaidya [1,3], Hirohiko Kakizaki [1] and Yasuhiro Takahashi [1,*]

[1] Department of Oculoplastic, Orbital & Lacrimal Surgery, Aichi Medical University Hospital, Nagakute 480-1195, Aichi, Japan; steffsomeda@gmail.com (S.K.S.); nume0828@yahoo.co.jp (N.U.); aricvaidya1@gmail.com (A.V.); cosme_geka@yahoo.co.jp (H.K.)
[2] Department of Ophthalmology, Aichi Medical University, Nagakute 480-1195, Aichi, Japan
[3] Department of Oculoplastic, Orbital & Lacrimal Surgery, Kirtipur Eye Hospital, Kathmandu 44600, Nepal
* Correspondence: yasuhiro_tak@yahoo.co.jp; Tel.: +81-561-62-3311 (ext. 12314)

Abstract: This retrospective, observational study examined the surgical outcomes of bilateral inferior rectus (IR) recession in thyroid eye disease. Twelve patients who underwent bilateral IR muscle recession were included in the study. Surgical success was defined as patient achievement of the following conditions: (1) a postoperative angle of vertical ocular deviation of $\leq 3°$; (2) a postoperative cyclotropic angle of $\leq 2°$; (3) postoperative binocular single vision, including the primary position; and (4) postoperative enlargement of the field of binocular single vision. Linear regression analyses were performed to analyze the relationship between postoperative changes in the vertical and torsional ocular deviation angles and the amount of IR muscle recession and nasal transposition. Consequently, 9 out of 12 patients were deemed to have had successful surgical outcomes. There was a positive correlation between a change in the vertical deviation angle and a side-related difference in the amount of IR muscle recession in successful cases (crude coefficient, 2.524). A positive correlation was also found between a change in the torsional deviation angle and the amount of IR recession (crude coefficient, 1.059) and nasal transposition (crude coefficient, 5.907). The results will be helpful to more precisely determine the amount of recession and nasal transposition of the IR muscle in patients with thyroid-related bilateral IR myopathy.

Keywords: bilateral inferior rectus muscle recession; nasal inferior rectus muscle transposition; restrictive strabismus; thyroid eye disease

Citation: Someda, S.K.; Umezawa, N.; Vaidya, A.; Kakizaki, H.; Takahashi, Y. Surgical Outcomes of Bilateral Inferior Rectus Muscle Recession for Restrictive Strabismus Secondary to Thyroid Eye Disease. *J. Clin. Med.* **2023**, *12*, 6876. https://doi.org/10.3390/jcm12216876

Academic Editor: Andrzej Grzybowski

Received: 5 September 2023
Revised: 25 October 2023
Accepted: 28 October 2023
Published: 31 October 2023

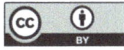

Copyright: © 2023 by the authors. Licensee MDPI, Basel, Switzerland. This article is an open access article distributed under the terms and conditions of the Creative Commons Attribution (CC BY) license (https://creativecommons.org/licenses/by/4.0/).

1. Introduction

Thyroid eye disease (TED) is a debilitating condition, with approximately 15% of patients with TED suffering from symptomatic ocular motility disturbance due to fibrotic changes in the extraocular muscles [1]. Among the extraocular muscles, the inferior rectus (IR) and medial rectus (MR) are known to be commonly affected. When an active inflammation has subsided and the IR muscle becomes fibrotic, patients often complain of intractable diplopia, especially for vertical and torsional ocular misalignments. This leads to difficulty in performing daily activities, such as driving, reading, writing, and eating, thus affecting the quality of life in many patients. Patients elevate their chins and tilt their heads in order to compensate for vertical and torsional diplopia, while patients with severe vertical and torsional strabismus cannot obtain binocular single vision, despite compensatory head positioning or even spectacle correction using prism glasses [2]. The primary goal of strabismus surgery in patients with inactive TED is to achieve a substantial field of binocular single vision (BSV) in the primary, as well as in the downward, position [3–5]. However, the surgical outcomes of strabismus surgery in TED can be highly unpredictable, with 17% to 45% of cases requiring reoperation due to undercorrection, overcorrection, and postoperative torsional deviations [1,4,6]. One of the possible reasons for unpredictable surgical outcomes is the variation in the degree of fibrous changes and adipose degeneration in the extraocular muscles among patients with TED [2,7].

Bilateral IR myopathy is a relatively common condition associated with TED. In such cases, the bilateral restriction of supraduction and a large angle of excyclotropia make it more difficult to obtain BSV in any gaze direction [8]. Although IR muscle recession is usually performed to correct this condition, unilateral muscle surgery (only on the more severe eye) can cause progressive overcorrection due to increased stimulation in the contralateral superior rectus (SR) muscle, resulting in hypertropia of the ipsilateral eye, which can be explained by Hering's law [6,8,9]. Sprunger and Helveston indicated that half of the patients with TED who underwent unilateral IR recession experienced progressive overcorrection [9]. Therefore, asymmetric bilateral IR muscle recession is a better option to overcome this problem. However, since the IR muscle is a secondary adductor [10], bilateral IR muscle recession occasionally leads to an A-pattern strabismus [11,12]. Dagi et al. determined that postoperative A-pattern strabismus was found when the IR was recessed more than 6 mm [4]. This is due to the recruitment of the superior oblique (SO) muscle during infraduction or the possibility of excessive SO tone. On the other hand, Jellema et al. claimed that their study revealed no real A-pattern postoperatively, but mentioned the presence of a reduced horizontal squint angle, especially in the downward (primary position, 1.0°; downward, 3.0°) [13].

In the past, there have been few reports regarding the surgical outcomes of bilateral IR recession in TED [1,6,8,13–15]. The surgical outcomes of bilateral IR muscle recession reported in these previous reports were favorable, with surgical success rates of 64–100%. However, most of these reports included either a small number of patients (3–8 patients) [1,6,8,14] or patients with a prior history of orbital decompression [1,13,15], which causes further restriction of extraocular muscle motility [16,17]. To date, only one published report investigated the factors affecting the surgical outcomes of bilateral IR muscle recession [13]. This report presented the dose–effect relationship between improved elevation and the amount of IR muscle recession. Although improvement in supraduction is a good outcome measurement, the deviation angle in the primary position would be a more important postoperative finding of strabismus surgery in TED because obtaining a substantial field of BSV in the primary position is indeed the primary goal in these cases. None of the previous studies determined the relationship between the changes in ocular deviation angles in the primary position and the amount of IR muscle recession and nasal transposition. Understanding this relationship will ensure a more tailored bilateral IR muscle recession for TED patients [2,7]. We have conducted this study to determine the effectiveness of asymmetric bilateral IR recession for the management of restrictive strabismus in patients diagnosed with TED who did not undergo orbital decompression.

2. Materials and Methods

2.1. Ethics Approval

The institutional review board (IRB) of Aichi Medical University Hospital approved this study, which was conducted in accordance with the tenets of the Declaration of Helsinki and its later amendments (approval number, 2023-022). The IRB granted a waiver of informed consent for this study, based on the ethical guidelines for medical and health research involving human subjects established by the Japanese Ministry of Education, Culture, Sports, Science, and Technology, and by the Ministry of Health, Labor, and Welfare. The waiver was granted because the study was a retrospective chart review, not an interventional study. Nevertheless, at the request of the IRB, an outline of the study, available for public viewing, was published on the Aichi Medical University website, which also gave the patients an option to refuse to participate in the study, although none of the patients did. Personal identifiers were removed from the records prior to data analysis.

2.2. Study Design

This retrospective, observational study included Japanese patients with TED who underwent asymmetric bilateral IR muscle recession, with or without IR muscle nasal transposition, at Aichi Medical University Hospital, Japan, performed by one of the authors (Y.T.) from January 2015 to February 2023. The restriction of upward gaze was graded on an ordinal scale (0 = duction > 45°, 1 = 30–45°, 2 = 15–30°, and 3 = <15°) [18,19], and patients with at least grade 1 in a less severe eye were included in this study. Bilateral positive forced duction tests were confirmed intraoperatively in all patients. Patients with a lack of clinical data, a history of strabismus or orbital decompression surgery, a follow-up period of less than 3 months, concomitant neuro-ophthalmologic disorder(s), and an intracranial lesion were excluded from this study. Since the outcome and its associated changes were best measured after a certain duration of follow-up from the time of surgical intervention, a retrospective, observational approach was deemed appropriate for this study.

2.3. Diagnosis of TED

A diagnosis of TED was based on the presence of at least one of the characteristic eyelid signs (eyelid fullness, eyelid retraction, and/or eyelid lag), as well as the presence of elevated thyroid antibody levels [10]. All patients included in this study were diagnosed with an autoimmune thyroid disorder by their endocrinologists prior to referral to our service. The IR muscle was confirmed to be enlarged, without muscle tendon involvement, on magnetic resonance images (MRI), and upward gaze was restricted on both sides in all patients, which also supported the diagnosis of TED. All patients included in the study were controlled as euthyroid at the time of surgery. We confirmed that all patients were in the static or chronic "burnout" phase of TED, based on the clinical activity score of 0 to 1 immediately before surgery and the absence of inflammation in the extraocular muscles on T2-weighted fat-suppressed MRIs obtained 3 months prior to the surgery.

2.4. Data Collection

The charts of all TED patients who underwent asymmetric bilateral IR recession surgery were reviewed from the electronic medical record (EMR) of the hospital. The following data from the EMR were collected: age, sex, smoking status, history of steroid pulse therapy and/or orbital radiotherapy, amounts of IR muscle recession and nasal IR muscle transposition, concomitant strabismus surgery, preoperative and postoperative angles of ocular deviation, and preoperative and postoperative fields of BSV. We asked all the patients the number of cigarettes smoked per day. Patients who previously smoked but stopped smoking cigarettes ≥2 years prior to the examinations were considered non-smokers [20]. The smoking status was classified by the number of cigarettes smoked per day, according to a report by Pfeilschifter and Ziegler, as follows: 0, no smoking; 1, <10 cigarettes/day; 2, 10–20 cigarettes/day; and 3, >20 cigarettes/day [21]. The dose used for orbital radiotherapy was 20 Gy in all the treated patients.

Preoperative and postoperative measurements of ocular deviation angles and the field of BSV were carried out by an exclusive orthoptist (N.U.) one day before and three months after surgery, respectively. The angle of ocular deviation was measured using a synoptophore (Clement Clarke International Ltd., Edinburgh, UK). The patient's head was positioned upright, and the instrument was set such that the fixating eye was the eye on which surgery was planned. One of the two arms of the synoptophore was fixed at 0°. We used two slides: a black circle with a cross-shaped blank and a black cross (L-25G; Inami, Tokyo, Japan). The black circle slide was fixed in the arm of the fixating eye, and the patient was asked to move the black cross until it was positioned appropriately within the circle. We then recorded the angle at which this was achieved. The deviation angles were measured in the primary position, at the 15° upward gaze, and at the 15° downward gaze. The Goldmann perimeter (Haag Streit, Bern, Switzerland) was used to measure the field of BSV.

The areas of fields of BSV were measured using the freehand measuring tool available in ImageJ software ver. 1.49 (National Institute of Health, Bethesda, MD, USA). We first measured the normal area of BSV in Japanese, based on our previous study [22], and then determined the areas of pre- and postoperative fields of BSV (Figure 1). The percentages of pre- and postoperative fields of BSV were calculated against the normal field of BSV (%BSV). In addition, the results of the field of BSV were classified into five categories (B1 to B5), according to the methods used in our previous study [23], as follows: B1, within normal range ($\pm 2 \times$ standard deviations); B2, the field of BSV reaches at least 20 degrees superiorly, 40 degrees inferiorly, and 30 degrees horizontally; B3, the field of BSV is smaller than that of B2, but includes primary gaze; B4, the field of BSV does not include primary gaze; B5, the field of BSV cannot be obtained in any direction of gaze.

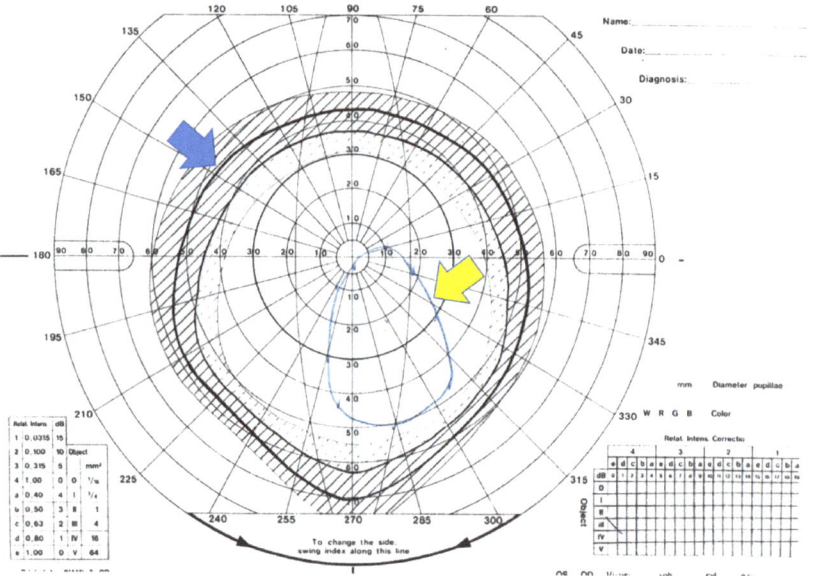

Figure 1. Measurements of normal (blue arrow) and actual (yellow arrow) fields of binocular single vision (BSV). Dashed shaded area means the range of ±1 standard deviation value of the measurement results of the field of BSV in normal Japanese volunteers [22]. Dotted area means there is a range of −2 standard deviation value.

2.5. MRI

MRI was performed using a 1.5-Tesla scanner (Magnetom Abant™; Siemens Healthcare, Erlangen, Germany), with the patients in the supine position. Coronal T1- and T2-weighted gradient-echo sequences were acquired (T1—repetition time: 500 ms, echo time: 10 ms, field of view: 140 × 140 mm, matrix: 256 × 220, section thickness: 3 mm with a 0.6 mm gap between slices; T2—repetition time: 4000 ms, echo time: 100 ms; all other parameters were the same as in T1). Patients were asked to look at a light source to ensure that their eyes were fixed in the primary position. The cross-sectional areas of the IR, SR, MR, and SO muscles on a coronal T1-weighted MRI image and those of the lateral rectus muscle on an axial T1-weighted MRI image at the largest point were measured by one of the authors (Y.T.), using the measuring tool available in the MRI viewer (ShadeQuest/ViewR™; Yokogawa Medical Solutions Corporation, Tokyo, Japan) (Figure 2) [24]. This study did not measure the cross-sectional area of the inferior oblique muscle because sagittal images could not be obtained from some of the patients [25].

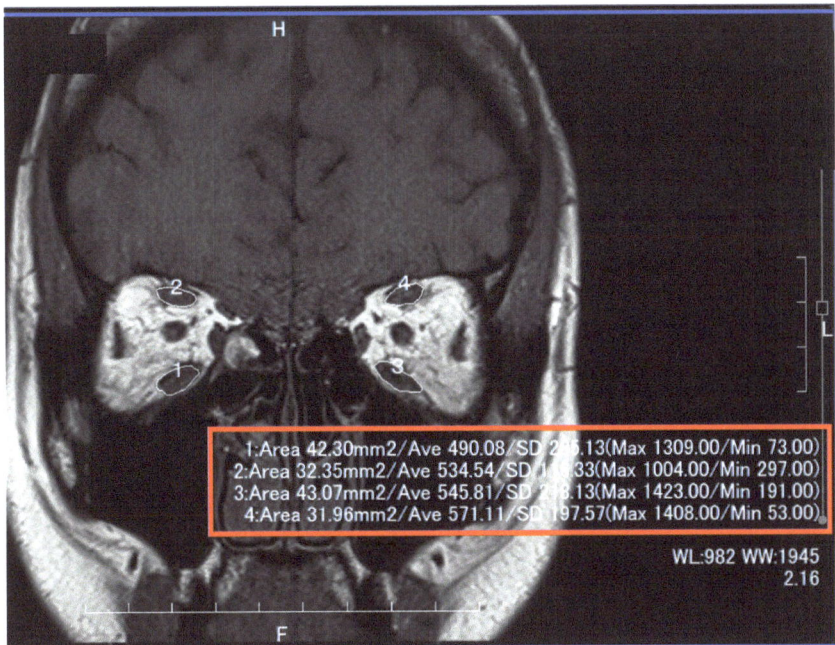

Figure 2. Measurements of the cross-sectional areas of inferior (#1 and #3) and superior (#2 and #4) recti muscles.

2.6. Surgical Procedure

Surgery was performed under general anesthesia using the same method of IR muscle recession employed in our previous studies [2,7,10]. A perilimbal conjunctival incision, with radial relaxing incisions, was made in the inferior or inferonasal quadrant. A muscle hook was used to secure the IR muscle at its insertion, and the Tenon's capsule around the IR muscle was thoroughly dissected using cotton swabs. The width of the IR muscle tendon was measured at the scleral insertion using a caliper. The IR muscle tendon was secured using locking 6-0 or 8-0 polyglactin sutures (Vicryl®; Johnson and Johnson Company, New Brunswick, NJ, USA) at two points 1 mm posterior to the globe insertion because of the 1 mm tip thickness of the muscle hook. Then, the IR muscle was detached from its insertion. The sutures were fixed to the sclera 1 mm posterior to the point that was estimated based on the preoperative angle of the vertical ocular deviation and the grade of upward gaze restriction. More hypotropic eyes with a more severe restriction of supraduction were defined as more severe eyes. The maximum amount of IR recession in a more severe eye was set at 8 mm [26,27]. The amount of IR recession in a less severe eye was commonly set at 3 mm [1]. In patients with grade 1 in a less severe eye, it was set at 2 mm. The recession of the IR muscle in a more severe eye was calculated, based on the following formula: 2° of hypotropic angle per 1 mm IR muscle recession + the amount of IR recession in a less severe eye [7]. When patients were aware of torsional diplopia before surgery and when the preoperative excyclotropia angle was larger than the estimated excyclotropic angle correction after the inferior rectus muscle, calculated with the undermentioned formula, we transposed the IR muscle nasally along the spiral of Tillaux. The amount of nasal IR muscle transposition was preoperatively calculated based on the preoperative angle of excyclotropia and the measurement result of the tendon width as follows: 8° of excyclotropic angle per one IR muscle tendon width transposition +0.4° of excyclotropic angle per 1 mm IR muscle recession [2]. In anticipation of late overcorrection, we set the target angles of the vertical and torsional deviations with the remaining 2–3° of hypotropia and 1–2° of excyclotropia. The IR muscle tendon was additionally fixed to the sclera using

6-0 or 8-0 polyglactin sutures at two to four points to prevent the slippage of the muscle. Finally, the conjunctiva was closed using 8-0 polyglactin sutures.

2.7. Statistical Analyses

Patient data and measurement results were expressed as the means ± standard deviations. To evaluate the pattern strabismus, the horizontal deviation angle measured in a 15° downward gaze was subtracted from that measured in a 15° upward gaze. The values were expressed as positive and negative for the tendency of A- and V-pattern strabismus, respectively. As we roughly set the measurement of two prism diopters corresponding to 1°, subtraction values of 5° and −7.5° or greater were considered to indicate clinically significant A- and V-pattern strabismus, respectively [28]. Surgical success was defined as patient achievement of the following four conditions: (1) a postoperative angle of vertical ocular deviation of ≤3°; (2) a postoperative cyclotropic angle of ≤2°; (3) a postoperative BSV grade of B3 or better; and (4) postoperative improvement of %BSV. Comparisons of patient age, ratio of patients with history of steroid pulse therapy/orbital radiotherapy, ratio of smoking status, amount of IR muscle recession and nasal transposition, ratio of patients who underwent additional strabismus surgery, cross-sectional areas of the extraocular muscles in more and less severe eyes, preoperative ocular deviation angles, preoperative pattern strabismus, and preoperative BSV grade between the successful and unsuccessful groups were conducted via the Mann–Whitney U test, Fisher's exact test, or the Chi-square test. Due to the small sample size, the Mann–Whitney U test and Fisher's exact test were used for the comparison of independent samples and the analyses of 2 × 2 tables, respectively, rather than the Student's t-test or the Chi-square test. Univariate linear regression analysis was performed to analyze the relationship between the side-related difference in the amount of IR muscle recession and the postoperative changes in the vertical ocular deviation angle. Univariate and subsequent multivariate linear regression analyses, with stepwise variable selection, were performed to identify factors influencing changes in torsional deviation angles. The predictive variables investigated included the amount of IR muscle nasal transposition in both more and less severe eyes and the sum of the amount of IR muscle recession in both eyes. We conducted linear regression analyses in all cases. All statistical analyses were performed using SPSS™ version 26 software (IBM Japan, Tokyo, Japan). Two-tailed p values < 0.05 were deemed to indicate statistical significance.

3. Results

Data regarding patient characteristics, surgery, and measurements are shown in Table 1. This study included 12 patients (2 males and 10 females; patient age, 60.6 ± 8.6 years). Six patients exhibited more severe right eyes, while six patients possessed more severe left eyes.

The amount of IR recession was 6.1 ± 1.7 mm in the more severe eyes. In the less severe eyes, the amount of IR recession was set at 2 mm in 2 patients and at 3 mm in 10 patients. The side-related difference in the amount of IR recession was 3.3 ± 1.5 mm. The amount of IR muscle nasal transposition was 0.2 ± 0.3 muscle width in more severe eyes and 0.1 ± 0.1 muscle width in less severe eyes. Bilateral and unilateral (more severe eyes) IR muscle nasal transpositions were performed in 2 and 3 patients, respectively, while the other 7 patients did not undergo nasal transposition of the IR muscle. Bilateral and unilateral MR muscle recession was performed in 1 and 2 patients, respectively, for correction of concomitant esotropia.

The surgical outcomes are shown in Table 2. Before surgery, the angles of hypotropia, esotropia, excyclotropia, and pattern deviation were 6.2 ± 3.8°, 6.0 ± 5.3°, 5.4 ± 3.7°, and 0.8 ± 3.8°, respectively. A-pattern strabismus was present in 3 patients. Preoperative %BSV was 19.6 ± 21.4%, and preoperative BSV grade was B3 in 4 patients, B4 in 4 patients, and B5 in 4 patients, respectively. After surgery, the angles of hypotropia, esotropia, excyclotropia, and pattern deviation decreased to 2.3 ± 3.6°, 1.0 ± 3.2°, −0.1 ± 1.4°, and −0.5 ± 3.0°, respectively. A-pattern strabismus was corrected after bilateral IR muscle recession, without nasal transposition, in the 3 patients due to a greater reduction of the horizontal deviation angle in the upward gaze compared to that in downward gaze. None of the patients with A-pattern strabismus exhibited incyclotropia before or after surgery. None of the other 9 patients developed new-onset pattern strabismus. Postoperatively, the %BSV increased to 45.5 ± 26.3%, and the BSV grade was B1 in 1 patient, B2 in 5 patients, B3 in 3 patients, and B4 in 3 patients.

Table 1. Data for patient characteristics, surgery, and measurement results.

	Total	Successful	Unsuccessful	p Value
Patient number	12	9	3	
M/F	2/10	2/7	0/3	1.000
Patient age (years) (range)	60.6 ± 8.6 (45–75)	59.6 ± 9.4 (45–75)	63.7 ± 5.7 (59–70)	0.373
History of steroid pulse/orbital radiation therapies (Y/N)	8/4	7/2	1/2	0.236
Smoking status				
Non-smoker	9	7	2	0.157
<10 cigarettes/day	0	0	0	
11–20 cigarettes/day	2	2	0	
>20 cigarettes/day	1	0	1	
More severe eyes (R/L)	6/6	5/5	1/2	
Amount of IR muscle recession in more severe eyes (mm) (range)	6.1 ± 1.7 (3.0–8.0)	5.7 ± 1.8 (3.0–8.0)	7.3 ± 1.2 (6.0–8.0)	0.209
Amount of IR muscle recession in less severe eyes				
2 mm	2	2	0	1.000
3 mm	10	7	3	
Side-related difference in amount of IR muscle recession (mm) (range)	3.3 ± 1.5 (1.0–5.0)	2.9 ± 1.5 (1.0–5.0)	4.3 ± 1.2 (3.0–5.0)	0.209
Amount of IR muscle nasal transposition (muscle width) (range)				
More severe eyes	0.2 ± 0.3 (0–1.0)	0.2 ± 0.3 (0–0.5)	0.3 ± 0.6 (0–1.0)	1.000
Less severe eyes	0.1 ± 0.1 (0–0.3)	0.1 ± 0.1 (0–0.3)	0.1 ± 0.2 (0–0.3)	0.600
Additional treatment				
Unilateral MR muscle recession	2	1	1	0.595
Bilateral MR muscle recession	1	1	0	
Cross-sectional area of IR muscle (mm^2) (range)				
More severe eyes	64.8 ± 15.7 (42.3–101.3)	61.5 ± 12.2 (42.3–77.3)	74.5 ± 23.7 (56.3–101.3)	0.727
Less severe eyes	61.1 ± 15.6 (41.3–86.5)	61.6 ± 15.9 (41.3–86.5)	59.8 ± 17.7 (43.5–78.6)	1.000
Cross-sectional area of SR muscle (mm^2) (range)				
More severe eyes	27.4 ± 7.5 (10.0–36.2)	28.1 ± 5.3 (19.6–35.6)	25.3 ± 13.7 (10.0–36.2)	0.864
Less severe eyes	31.6 ± 10.0 (12.6–47.7)	32.6 ± 9.0 (20.7–47.7)	28.4 ± 14.3 (12.6–40.2)	1.000
Cross-sectional area of MR muscle (mm^2) (range)				
More severe eyes	41.1 ± 8.6 (30.5–60.8)	39.6 ± 5.9 (33.9–49.8)	45.7 ± 15.1 (30.5–60.8)	0.727
Less severe eyes	42.2 ± 7.7 (34.0–56.3)	41.7 ± 7.1 (34.0–54.6)	43.8 ± 10.8 (36.6–56.3)	0.727

Table 1. Cont.

Cross-sectional area of SO muscle (mm²) (range)					
	More severe eyes	17.0 ± 6.9 (8.4–30.9)	17.2 ± 5.0 (12.3–26.3)	16.3 ± 12.7 (8.4–30.9)	0.482
	Less severe eyes	17.4 ± 4.2 (12.0–26.8)	17.0 ± 4.5 (12.0–26.8)	18.7 ± 3.9 (14.5–22.3)	0.482
Cross-sectional area of LR muscle (mm²) (range)					
	More severe eyes	130.0 ± 29.8 (80.0–165.8)	132.4 ± 28.5 (80.0–165.8)	122.5 ± 39.3 (82.6–161.0)	0.864
	Less severe eyes	127.6 ± 31.7 (84.8–167.3)	128.6 ± 31.0 (84.8–164.8)	125.5 ± 40.9 (85.6–167.3)	1.000

M, male; F, female; Y, yes; N, no; R, right; L, left; IR, inferior rectus; MR, medial rectus; SR, superior rectus; MR, medial rectus; SO, superior oblique; LR, lateral rectus.

A comparison of successful and unsuccessful cases is shown in Tables 1 and 3. Nine patients (75.0%) were deemed as successful surgical cases. The other 3 patients were considered unsuccessful cases due to the undercorrection of hypotropia. In 2 of these 3 cases, excyclotropia was adequately corrected, but the other 1 case showed the overcorrection of excyclotropia (−4 degrees). Although none of the measurements were significantly different based on statistical analysis, the amount of IR recession in more severe eyes seemed to be larger in unsuccessful cases (5.7 ± 1.8 mm vs. 7.3 ± 1.2 mm; $p = 0.209$). Additional SR muscle surgery was performed in the 3 unsuccessful cases, after which all the 3 cases obtained a field of BSV of B3 or better.

Table 2. Surgical outcomes.

		Preoperative	Postoperative
Ocular deviation angle (degrees) (range)			
	Hypotropia	6.2 ± 3.8 (1–13)	2.3 ± 3.6 (−1–10)
	Esotropia	6.0 ± 5.3 (0–15)	1.0 ± 3.2 (−7–6)
	Excyclotropia	5.4 ± 3.7 (1–15)	−0.1 ± 1.4 (−4–2)
	Magnitude of pattern strabismus	0.8 ± 3.8 (−5–6)	−0.5 ± 3.0 (−7–4)
Pattern strabismus			
	A-pattern	3	0
	V-pattern	0	0
%BSV (%)		19.6 ± 21.4 (0–56.4)	45.5 ± 26.3 (9.0–86.0)
Grade of BSV			
	B1	0	1
	B2	0	5
	B3	4	3
	B4	4	3
	B5	4	0

BSV, binocular single vision.

Table 3. Comparison of surgical outcomes between successful and unsuccessful cases.

	Successful (n = 9)		Unsuccessful (n = 3)			p Value: vs. Preoperative Values
	Preoperative	Postoperative	Preoperative	Postoperative	After Additional Surgery	
Ocular deviation angle (degrees) (range)						
Hypotropia	5.8 ± 3.9 (0–13)	0.3 ± 0.7 (−1–1)	7.3 ± 4.0 (3–11)	8.0 ± 1.7 (7–10)	2.0 ± 1.7 (1–4)	0.727
Esotropia	6.0 ± 5.5 (0–15)	1.8 ± 2.2 (−1–6)	6.0 ± 5.6 (1–12)	−1.3 ± 4.9 (−7–2)	1.0 ± 2.6 (−2–3)	0.864
Excyclotropia	4.4 ± 2.4 (1–9)	0.2 ± 0.7 (0–2)	8.3 ± 5.8 (5–15)	−1.0 ± 2.6 (−4–1)	0 ± 1.7 (−2–1)	0.282
Magnitude of pattern strabismus	0.8 ± 4.0 (−5–6)	−0.9 ± 3.0 (−7–2)	0.7 ± 3.8 (−2–5)	0.7 ± 3.5 (−3–4)		1.000
Pattern strabismus						
A-pattern	2	0	1	0		0.491
V-pattern	0	0	0	0		
%BSV (%)	20.9 ± 24.1 (0–56.4)	55.7 ± 21.5 (25.3–86.0)	15.9 ± 12.9 (1.0–24.1)	14.8 ± 7.9 (9.0–23.8)	43.5 ± 16.5 (31.2–62.2)	0.727
Grade of BSV						
B1	0	1	0	0	0	
B2	0	5	0	0	1	
B3	3	3	1	0	2	0.449
B4	2	0	2	3	0	
B5	4	0	0	0	0	

BSV, binocular single vision.

The results of the linear regression analyses are shown in Table 4. Univariate analysis for the correction of hypotropia showed that, although the change in the vertical ocular deviation angle was not correlated with the side-related difference in the total amount of IR muscle recession ($p = 0.125$), there was a correlation between the side-related difference and the amount of IR muscle recession in successful cases ($p < 0.001$) (adjusted $R^2 = 0.923$; $p < 0.001$). The crude coefficient of the side-related difference in the amount of IR muscle recession was 2.524. Multivariate stepwise analysis showed that the change in the cyclotropic angle was correlated with the amount of IR nasal transposition in more severe eyes ($p = 0.012$) and the sum of the total amount of IR muscle recession ($p = 0.005$) (adjusted $R^2 = 0.817$; $p < 0.001$). The crude coefficients of the amount of IR muscle nasal transposition in more severe eyes and the sum of the amount of IR muscle recession were 5.907 and 1.059, respectively. Multivariate stepwise analysis also showed that a change in the cyclotropic angle was correlated with the sum of the amount of IR muscle recession ($p = 0.006$) in successful cases (adjusted $R^2 = 0.689$; $p = 0.006$). The crude coefficient of the sum of the amount of IR muscle recession was 1.000.

Table 4. Results of univariate and multivariate analyses.

Changes in Vertical Ocular Deviation Angle	Univariate					
Total	p Value	Crude Coefficient	95% CI			
Side-related difference in amount of IR muscle recession	0.125	1.548	−0.513 to 3.610			
Successful cases						
Side-related difference in amount of IR muscle recession	<0.001	2.524	1.874 to 3.173			
Changes in torsional angle	Univariate			Multivariate		
Total	p value	Crude coefficient	95% CI	p value	Crude coefficient	95% CI
Amount of nasal transposition of IR muscle in more severe eyes	0.007	8.788	3.017 to 14.559	0.012	5.907	1.661 to 10.153
Amount of nasal transposition of IR muscle in less severe eyes	0.004	21.818	8.525 to 35.111			
Sum of amount of IR muscle recession	0.002	1.427	0.634 to 2.220	0.005	1.059	0.417 to 1.702
Successful cases						
Amount of nasal transposition of IR muscle in more severe eyes	0.072	8.069	−0.936 to 17.074			
Amount of nasal transposition of IR muscle in less severe eyes	0.034	16.288	1.676 to 30.900			
Sum of amount of IR muscle recession	0.006	1.000	0.339 to 1.601	0.006	1.000	0.339 to 1.601

IR, inferior rectus; CI, confidence interval.

4. Discussion

This study investigated the surgical outcomes of bilateral asymmetric IR recession in TED and the factors influencing them. Surgical success was obtained in 75% of patients in our study. Cruz and Davitt reported that six out of eight patients were found to have successful correction of hypotropia, while the other two patients remained undercorrected [6]. Flanders and Hastings presented their surgical outcomes, with all three patients obtaining complete correction of hypotropia, but one of the three patients underwent symmetric IR recession [14]. Another patient underwent a second surgery, but the amount of IR recession was not mentioned [14]. Arnolds and Reynolds reported their surgical outcomes, with all four patients deemed as surgical success, but the detailed surgical methods were not presented [8]. In the report by Jellema et al., 64% of patients required no further surgery after bilateral IR muscle recession, while 17% of patients needed one or more additional vertical strabismus surgeries [13]. Volpe et al. demonstrated that 45 out of 54 patients (84%) obtained a final vertical deviation angle of <5 prism diopters, but they combined patients who underwent unilateral and bilateral IR muscle recession ± contralateral SR muscle recession [1]. The surgical outcomes of our study were comparable to those of the aforementioned studies.

Previous studies have reported that an enlarged SR muscle can cause failure of bilateral IR muscle recession due to underestimation of excyclotorsion and late overcorrection of hypotropia [4–6,8]. Although there were three unsuccessful cases in this study, those three patients showed that the undercorrection of hypotropia and the cross-sectional areas of the SR muscle in both eyes were not significantly different between the successful and unsuccessful cases. The difference may not have been statistically significant, but the amount of IR recession in the more severe eyes seemed to be larger in the unsuccessful cases (5.7 ± 1.8 mm vs. 7.3 ± 1.2 mm). A large amount of IR recession in the more severe eye may cause divergence between the expected and actual dose–effect response of bilateral IR muscle recession.

The change in the vertical ocular deviation angle was correlated with the side-related difference in the amount of IR muscle recession in the successful cases, and the crude coefficient of the side-related difference was 2.524. This means that for every 1 mm of difference in the amount of IR recession between the right and left eyes, there are 2.524 degrees of hypotropia improvement in the more severe eye. This coefficient was close to the one reported in our previous study, showing the mean dose–effect relationship of unilateral IR muscle recession to be 2.27 ± 0.6 degrees/mm [7]. Jellema et al. further reported on the surgical outcomes of bilateral IR muscle recession, showing the dose–effect response to be $1.7 \pm 1.7°$ for every millimeter of recession [13]. However, since this dose–effect response was only noted for improved elevation, it was not comparable with the coefficient shown in our study. Moreover, Jellema's report included patients with a prior history of orbital decompression.

The change in torsional angle was correlated with the amount of IR nasal transposition in the more severe eyes (crude coefficient of 5.907), which was notably smaller compared to that in our previous study showing the results of unilateral IR muscle recession and nasal transposition in TED (crude coefficient of 8.546) [2]. On the other hand, the correlation of the torsional angle change and the sum of the amount of IR muscle recession (crude coefficient of 1.059) seemed to be larger than the coefficient derived from unilateral IR muscle recession (crude coefficient of 0.405) reported in our previous study [2]. In this present study, the amount of IR muscle nasal transposition was preoperatively calculated based on the result of unilateral IR muscle recession shown in our previous study, which was 8° of excyclotropic angle per one IR muscle tendon width transposition + 0.4° of excyclotropic angle per millimeter of IR muscle recession [2]. However, the results of unilateral IR muscle recession and nasal transposition cannot be applied to patients who require bilateral IR muscle recession. The study by Jellema et al. also showed improvement in the squint angle with regards to primary gaze, as well as reduced excyclotorsion, with a dose–effect response of $0.74 \pm 0.61°$ per millimeter of recession in the primary position, postoperatively [13]. This value was relatively intermediate between the values shown in the present study and those in our previous study [2].

Three patients exhibited A-pattern strabismus before surgery, which was corrected after bilateral IR recession, without IR nasal transposition. In addition, none of the other nine patients experienced new-onset pattern strabismus after surgery. Kushner, in his study involving 51 patients with symptomatic diplopia on downward gaze at near vision, claimed that bilateral IR muscle recession in TED poses the risk of A-pattern strabismus and nasal transposition of the recessed IR muscle, as the prevention of A-pattern exotropia would aggravate incyclotropia [11]. However, since our previous study indicated that unilateral IR muscle recession ± IR nasal transposition does not increase the risk of pattern strabismus [10], the same conclusion may be applicable to bilateral IR muscle recession. There were no sources explaining the resolution of A-pattern strabismus after IR recession without nasal transposition. Theoretically, however, the restriction of the fibrotic IR muscle could have been causing compensatory overaction of the antagonist SR muscle, resulting in incyclotorsion and/or adduction on elevation, and the weakening of the IR muscle eventually led to the resolution of the SR overaction as well. On the other hand, a previous study showed that a thicker IR muscle caused A-pattern strabismus after IR muscle recession in TED [15]. We compared the thickness of the IR muscle between cases with and without A-pattern strabismus. It was noted that the IR muscle in more severe eyes was thinner in cases with A-pattern strabismus ($p = 0.036$), although the thickness was not different between cases with and without A-pattern strabismus in less severe eyes ($p = 0.864$). This may also affect the improvement of A-pattern strabismus in our study. Furthermore, nasal transposition of the IR muscle has been proven beneficial, both to correct excyclotropia and to prevent A-pattern strabismus [13], and setting the target torsional angle to 1–2° of undercorrection may prevent aggravating the incyclotropia after surgery.

This study has some limitations, one of which is a relatively small sample size, with only 12 patients included in the analysis. A small sample size can limit the statistical power of the study and may not adequately represent the diverse characteristics and variations in TED. Another limitation of this study is the short follow-up period. Postoperative ocular deviation angles and BSV results were obtained after only 3 months. The authors recommend a larger sample size and a longer duration of follow-up to gather more data on the surgical outcomes, as well as to account for the presence of late overcorrection. A retrospective study with a 2-year follow-up period was found to confirm the presence of late overcorrection in TED patients who underwent unilateral IR muscle recession for restrictive strabismus [5]. Previous studies have shown that IR muscle recession can result to lower eyelid retraction [29,30]. There was no data regarding changes in the lower eyelid position after surgery, hence presenting another limitation of the study. Furthermore, the authors used an ordinal scale of 0 to 3 as the grading system for ocular motility restriction, instead of the usual 0 to 4. A more universal grading system should probably be adopted for consistency across all published literature.

5. Conclusions

This study investigated the surgical outcomes of asymmetric bilateral IR muscle recession in TED. A total of 9 out of 12 patients (75.0%) were judged as successful surgical cases and obtained the field of binocular single vision in the primary position. In contrast, a large amount of IR muscle recession in a more severe eye might be the cause of undercorrection of hypotropia in the three unsuccessful cases. The coefficients of the amount of IR muscle recession and IR nasal transposition were shown for the correction of hypotropia and excyclotropia. This study indicates that bilateral IR muscle recession ± nasal transposition of the IR muscle proved to be beneficial in TED patients with vertical and torsional ocular deviation caused by fibrosis of the IR muscle, which can lead to debilitating diplopia. The results of linear regression analyses in this study will be helpful to more precisely determine the amount of IR muscle recession and IR nasal transposition required in TED patient with bilateral IR myopathy suffering from debilitating diplopia and to prevent the occurrence of postoperative ocular misalignments.

Author Contributions: Conceptualization, Y.T.; methodology, N.U. and Y.T.; validation, Y.T.; formal analysis, N.U. and Y.T.; investigation, N.U. and Y.T.; data curation, Y.T.; writing—original draft preparation, S.K.S.; writing—review and editing, N.U., A.V., H.K. and Y.T.; supervision, Y.T.; project administration, Y.T. All authors have read and agreed to the published version of the manuscript.

Funding: This research received no external funding.

Institutional Review Board Statement: The study was conducted in accordance with the Declaration of Helsinki, and approved by the Institutional Review Board of Aichi Medical University Hospital (approval number, 2023-022; date of approval, 15 June 2023).

Informed Consent Statement: Patient consent was waived due to the nature of the study as a retrospective chart review, not an interventional study, based on the ethical guidelines for medical and health research involving human subjects established by the Japanese Ministry of Education, Culture, Sports, Science, and Technology, and by the Ministry of Health, Labor, and Welfare. Personal identifiers were removed from the records prior to data analysis.

Data Availability Statement: Data supporting the results of this study are available on request.

Conflicts of Interest: The authors declare no conflict of interest.

References

1. Volpe, N.J.; Mirza-George, N.; Binenbaum, G. Surgical management of vertical ocular misalignment in thyroid eye disease using an adjustable suture technique. *J. AAPOS* **2012**, *16*, 518–522. [CrossRef] [PubMed]
2. Takahashi, Y.; Kitaguchi, Y.; Nakakura, S.; Mito, H.; Kimura, A.; Kakizaki, H. Correction of excyclotropia by surgery on the inferior rectus muscle in patients with thyroid eye disease: A retrospective, observational study. *PLoS ONE* **2016**, *11*, e0159562. [CrossRef] [PubMed]
3. Honglertnapakul, W.; Cavuoto, K.M.; McKeown, C.A.; Capó, H. Surgical treatment of strabismus in thyroid eye disease: Characteristics, dose-response, and outcomes. *J. AAPOS* **2020**, *24*, 72.e1–72.e7. [CrossRef] [PubMed]
4. Dagi, L.R. Understanding and managing vertical strabismus from thyroid eye disease. *J. AAPOS* **2018**, *22*, 252–255. [CrossRef]

5. Savino, G.; Mattei, R.; Salerni, A.; Fossataro, C.; Pafundi, P.C. Long-term follow-up of surgical treatment of thyroid-associated orbitopathy restrictive strabismus. *Front. Endocrinol.* **2022**, *13*, 1030422. [CrossRef]
6. Cruz, O.A.; Davitt, B.V. Bilateral inferior rectus muscle recession for correction of hypotonia in dysthyroid ophthalmopathy. *J. AAPOS* **1999**, *3*, 157–159. [CrossRef]
7. Takahashi, Y.; Kakizaki, H. Predictors of the dose-effect relationship regarding unilateral inferior rectus muscle recession in patients with thyroid eye disease. *Int. J. Endocrinol.* **2015**, *2015*, 703671. [CrossRef]
8. Arnoldi, K.; Reynolds, J.D. Unmasking bilateral inferior rectus restriction in thyroid eye disease: Using degree of cyclotropia. *Am. Orthopt. J.* **2015**, *65*, 81–86. [CrossRef]
9. Sprunger, D.T.; Helveston, E.M. Progressive overcorrection after inferior rectus recession. *J. Pediatr. Ophthalmol. Strabismus* **1993**, *30*, 145–148. [CrossRef]
10. Vaidya, A.; Kakizaki, H.; Takahashi, Y. Changes in horizontal strabismus after inferior rectus muscle recession with or without nasal transposition in thyroid eye disease: A retrospective, observational study. *PLoS ONE* **2020**, *15*, e0240019. [CrossRef]
11. Kushner, B.J. Management of diplopia limited to down gaze. *Arch. Ophthalmol.* **1995**, *113*, 1426–1430. [CrossRef] [PubMed]
12. Kushner, B.J. Torsion and pattern strabismus. *JAMA Ophthalmol.* **2013**, *131*, 190–193. [CrossRef]
13. Jellema, H.M.; Saeed, P.; Everhard-Halm, Y.; Prick, L.; Mourits, M. Bilateral inferior rectus muscle recession in patients with Graves orbitopathy: Is it effective? *Ophthalm. Plast. Reconstr. Surg.* **2012**, *28*, 268–272. [CrossRef] [PubMed]
14. Flanders, M.; Hastings, M. Diagnosis and surgical management of strabismus associated with thyroid-related orbitopathy. *J. Pediatr. Ophthalmol. Strabismus* **1997**, *34*, 333–340. [CrossRef] [PubMed]
15. Jellema, H.M.; Eckstein, A.; Oeverhaus, M.; Lacraru, I.; Saeed, P. Incidence of A pattern strabismus after inferior rectus recession in patients with Graves' orbitopathy: A retrospective multicentre study. *Acta. Ophthalmol.* **2023**, *101*, e106–e112. [CrossRef] [PubMed]
16. Eckstein, A.; Esser, J.; Oeverhaus, M.; Saeed, P.; Jellema, H.M. Surgical treatment of diplopia in Graves orbitopathy patients. *Ophthalmic. Plast. Reconstr. Surg.* **2018**, *34*, S75–S84. [CrossRef]
17. Gilbert, J.; Dailey, R.A.; Christensen, L.E. Characteristics and outcomes of strabismus surgery after orbital decompression surgery. *J. AAPOS* **2005**, *9*, 26–30. [CrossRef]
18. Barrio-Barrio, J.; Sabater, A.L.; Bonet-Farriol, E.; Velázquez-Villoria, Á.; Galofré, J.C. Graves' Ophthalmopathy: VISA versus EU-GOGO classification, assessment, and management. *J. Ophthalmol.* **2015**, *2015*, 249125. [CrossRef]
19. Karthiga, I. Extraocular movements. *Kerala. J. Ophthalmol.* **2020**, *32*, 209–212. [CrossRef]
20. Nunery, W.R.; Martin, R.T.; Heinz, G.W.; Gavin, T.J. The association of cigarette smoking with clinical subtypes of ophthalmic Graves' disease. *Ophthalmic. Plast. Reconstr. Surg.* **1993**, *9*, 77–82. [CrossRef]
21. Pfeilschifter, J.; Ziegler, R. Smoking and endocrine ophthalmopathy: Impact of smoking severity and current vs lifetime cigarette consumption. *Clin. Endocrinol.* **1996**, *45*, 477–481. [CrossRef]
22. Kakizaki, H.; Umezawa, N.; Takahashi, Y.; Selva, D. Binocular single vision field. *Ophthalmology* **2009**, *116*, 364. [CrossRef] [PubMed]
23. Takahashi, Y.; Sabundayo, M.S.; Miyazaki, H.; Mito, H.; Kakizaki, H. Orbital trapdoor fractures: Different clinical profiles between adult and paediatric patients. *Br. J. Ophthalmol.* **2018**, *102*, 885–891. [CrossRef] [PubMed]
24. Lee, P.A.L.; Vaidya, A.; Kono, S.; Kakizaki, H.; Takahashi, Y. Extraocular muscle expansion after deep lateral orbital wall decompression: Influence on proptosis reduction and its predictive factors. *Graefes. Arch. Clin. Exp. Ophthalmol.* **2021**, *259*, 3427–3435. [CrossRef] [PubMed]
25. Sabundayo, M.S.; Kakizaki, H.; Takahashi, Y. Normative measurements of inferior oblique muscle thickness in Japanese by magnetic resonance imaging using a new technique. *Graefes. Arch. Clin. Exp. Ophthalmol.* **2018**, *256*, 839–844. [CrossRef] [PubMed]
26. Esser, J.; Schittkowski, M.; Eckstein, A. Graves' orbitopaty: Inferior rectus tendon elongation for large vertical squint angles that cannot be corrected by simple muscle recession. *Klin. Monbl. Augenheilkd.* **2011**, *228*, 880–886. [CrossRef] [PubMed]
27. Oeverhaus, M.; Fischer, M.; Hirche, H.; Schlüter, A.; Esser, J.; Ecstein, A.K. Tendon elongation with bovine pericardium in patients with severe esotropia after decompression in Graves' orbitopathy-efficacy and long-term stability. *Strabismus* **2018**, *26*, 62–70. [CrossRef]
28. Straight, S.M.; Bahl, R.S. A- and V-pattern strabismus. In *Practical Management of Pediatric Ocular Disorders and Strabismus: A Case-Based Approach*; Traboulsi, E.I., Utz, V.M., Eds.; Springer: New York, NY, USA, 2016; pp. 583–584.
29. Norris, J.H.; Malhotra, R. Composite septo-retractor recession; a surgical technique for lower-eyelid retraction and review of the literature. *Ophthalmic. Plast. Reconstr. Surg.* **2011**, *27*, 447–452. [CrossRef]
30. Esser, J.; Ecstein, A. Ocular muscle and eyelid surgery in thyroid-associated orbitopathy. *Exp. Clin. Endocrinol. Diabetes* **1999**, *107* (Suppl. S5), S214–S221. [CrossRef]

Disclaimer/Publisher's Note: The statements, opinions and data contained in all publications are solely those of the individual author(s) and contributor(s) and not of MDPI and/or the editor(s). MDPI and/or the editor(s) disclaim responsibility for any injury to people or property resulting from any ideas, methods, instructions or products referred to in the content.

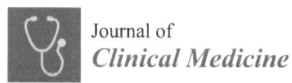

Article

Recovery of the Ratio of Closure Time during Blink Time in Lacrimal Passage Intubation

Yuri Kim and Helen Lew *

Department of Ophthalmology, Bundang CHA Medical Center, CHA University, Seongnam 13496, Republic of Korea; a206014@chamc.co.kr
* Correspondence: eye@cha.ac.kr; Tel.: +82-31-780-5330

Abstract: (1) Background: We aim to find a novel blink parameter in nasolacrimal duct obstruction (NDO) patients and analyze parameters that could reflect subjective symptoms and objective indicators at the same time through a blink dynamic analysis. (2) Methods A retrospective study was conducted with 34 patients (48 eyes) who underwent lacrimal passage intubation (LPI) and 24 control groups (48 eyes). All patients' blink patterns were measured using an ocular surface interferometer before and after LPI, including total blink (TB) and partial blink (PB) and the blink indices blink time (BT), lid closing time (LCT), closure time (CT), lid opening time (LOT), interblink time (IBT), closing speed (CS) and opening speed (OS). The tear meniscus height (TMH) was measured, and the questionnaire "Epiphora Patient's Quality of Life (E-QOL)," which includes daily activity restriction as well as static and dynamic activities, was completed. (3) Results: Compared to CT and the ratio of CT during BT (CT/BT) in control (89.4 ± 20.0 msec, 13.16%), those in NDOs were longer (140.3 ± 92.0 msec, 20.20%) and were also related to TMH. After LPI, CT and CT/BT were recovered to 85.4 ± 22.07 msec, 13.29% ($p < 0.001$). CT and CT/BT showed a positive correlation with the E-QOL questionnaire score, particularly with dynamic activities. (4) Conclusions: CT and CT/BT, which are objective indicators associated with subjective symptoms of patients, are considered new blink indices for the evaluation of NDO patients with Munk's score.

Keywords: blink index; ocular surface interferometer; nasolacrimal duct obstruction; closure time

Citation: Kim, Y.; Lew, H. Recovery of the Ratio of Closure Time during Blink Time in Lacrimal Passage Intubation. *J. Clin. Med.* **2023**, *12*, 3631. https://doi.org/10.3390/jcm12113631

Academic Editors: Kelvin Kam-Lung Chong, Renbing Jia and Maria Vittoria Cicinelli

Received: 8 March 2023
Revised: 30 March 2023
Accepted: 22 May 2023
Published: 23 May 2023

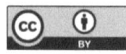

Copyright: © 2023 by the authors. Licensee MDPI, Basel, Switzerland. This article is an open access article distributed under the terms and conditions of the Creative Commons Attribution (CC BY) license (https://creativecommons.org/licenses/by/4.0/).

1. Introduction

There are two types of causes for epiphora: primary and secondary. Sung et al. developed the punctal reserve (PR) as a novel and clinically beneficial index for evaluating punctum parameters in nasolacrimal duct obstruction (NDO) patients using spectralis anterior segment optical coherence tomography (AS-OCT) scans [1].

There are various subjective ways for measuring the severity of epiphora, including Munk's score, the watery eye quality of life (WEQOL) questionnaire, and the TEARS (Times wiping eyes, Effects, Activities affected, Reflex tearing, Success) score [2,3]. The widely renowned Munk's score ranges from 0 to 5 and depicts the subjective discomfort of patients; however, there is a limit to just checking the daily numbers of wiping. To circumvent this constraint, the WEQOL questionnaire has been developed to assess the quality of life of epiphora patients [3]. The TEARS score gives a short and simple summary of the subjective and objective clinical severity of epiphora in patients, which can be utilized in a busy clinical setting [2]. TMH and PR are used to perform an objective evaluation of the amount of collected tears. Depending on the patient, the TMH and PR may objectively indicate the amount of collected tears, but further studies are necessary to investigate the subjective experiences of discomfort.

It is difficult to immediately detect subjective symptoms and objective indicators of tears due to the complexity of epiphora. Indicators that may simultaneously assess the subjective symptoms of patients and the objective parameters of epiphora are required for more precise diagnosis and evaluation.

NDO patients have a peculiar blinking pattern in which they squeeze their eyelids, and we attempted to identify novel indications by analyzing their blinking patterns. When NDO patients close their eyelids, they typically squeeze them as well. Thus, the pattern of their blinking is peculiar. By analyzing the blink pattern, we aimed to determine if it could be an additional diagnostic method of NDO.

A blink is an accurate reflection of the ocular surface and is related to the tear film's stability and the health of the ocular surface [4]. During a 20 s blink imaging analysis, blink patterns and blink dynamic indices were identified in blepharospasm, a facial nerve palsy [5,6]. In this study, we analyzed the link dynamic index for NDO patients using an ocular surface interferometer. In addition, we intended to identify important blink characteristics in NDO patients and assess how effectively subjective symptoms and objective indicators in NDO patients are reflected by indicators.

2. Materials and Methods

2.1. Participants

From July 2019 to January 2022, a retrospective study was performed on 34 patients (48 cases) who had lacrimal passage intubation (LPI), as well as 24 age- and gender-matched control groups (48 cases). To rule out other eyelid blinking effects, patients with a history of eyelid surgery, ocular disorders, and treatment were removed from the study. Although the relationship between dry eye disease symptoms and signs is weak and variable [7], individuals with dry eye disease were excluded. Age affects blinking [8]; thus, a retrospective study was conducted on 24 control groups (48 cases) with patients of similar ages and genders, with a mean age of 59.5 years in patients in their 40s and 60s who visited clinics for early cataract screening during medical visits.

2.2. Quality of Life in Epiphora Patients (E-QOL) Questionnaire

This is an E-QOL questionnaire utilized in this study that focuses on a patient's symptoms in addition to the Munk scale for patients who are currently visiting the outpatient clinic for epiphora. We identified subjective indicators that are more specific with regard to limitations on everyday living, static activities, and dynamic activities.

The total E-QOL questionnaire score was 60. The degree to which epiphora interferes with daily living was rated out of 10 points, whilst the degree to which it interferes with activities was rated out of 5 points. The daily activity limitation questionnaire has a score of 20 and consists of four questions: to what extent does tearing limit your daily activities? (0 = no limitations, 10 = severe limitations) To what extent does epiphora restrict your interpersonal relationships? (0 = no difficulty, 5 = constant difficulty) and how irritated are you owing to your tears? (0 = no trouble whatsoever, 5 = constant trouble). The static activity restriction questionnaire has a score of 25 and consists of five questions: how much difficulty do you have with reading, driving during the day, driving at night, using a computer, and watching television due to tearing? (0 = no trouble whatsoever, 5 = constant trouble). The dynamic activity restriction questionnaire has a score of 15 and consists of three questions: how much difficulty do you have with the following tasks at work, at home, and outside due to tearing?

2.3. Image Acquisition Method

Based on the 20 s videos (600 frames) captured using an ocular surface interferometer, the blink indices were analyzed. In the internal program of the ocular surface interferometer (LipiView®, TearScience Inc., Morrisville, NC, USA), the thickness of the lipid layer (LLT), total blink (TB, /20 s), and partial blink (PB, /20 s) were recorded. Spectralis anterior-segment OCT scans (AS-OCT, SPECTRALIS®, Heidelberg Engineering, GmbH, Heidelberg, Germany) were utilized to quantify tear meniscus height (TMH), punctal reserve (PR), and punctal diameter.

We define the blink cycle as the blink time (BT), which is the duration of the upper eyelid closing action, and the interblink time (IBT), which is the duration of the upper eyelid remaining open. BT was defined as the sum of the lid closing time (LCT—time taken by the interpalpebral fissure (IPF) to reach the maximum closure from the minimum closure), lid opening time (LOT—time taken by the upper eyelid to change from the minimum to maximum IPF), and closure time (CT—time that the upper eyelid remained completely closed).

Using these data, the blink index curve could be derived. For both the LCT and LOT periods, at least two time points were selected and calculated to determine the blink dynamic curve's curvature. Closing speed (CS) and opening speed (OS) were defined as the dynamic index of an eyelid's closure and opening, respectively. The CS and OS were computed using IPF per LCT (mm/s) and IPF per LOT (mm/s), respectively. The measurements were taken on all blinks that occurred within 20 s, and the results were averaged. The adjusted IPF versus time graph was used to generate each blink curve (Figure 1). For data gathering and analysis, a desktop computer running Windows 11 and video applications were utilized. Every measurement was taken by a single examiner (Y.K.).

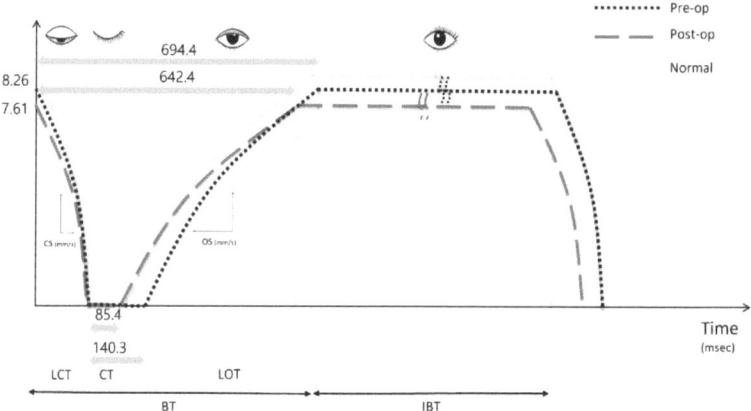

Figure 1. Blink indices graph of before and after lacrimal passage intubation (LPI) obtained using ocular surface interferometer (LipiView®). (BT, blink time; LCT, lid closing time; CT, closure time; LOT, lid opening time; IBT, interblink time; IPF, interpalpebral fissure; CS, closing speed; OS, opening speed).

The subjective satisfaction of patients following LPI whose TMH was less than 300 μm and who passed irrigation test were deemed successful.

2.4. Surgical Technique

As previously described, a single surgeon (H.L.) performed all of the procedures [9]. Using dacryoen doscopy and the insertion of a silicone tube, surgical treatment was performed under general or local anesthesia. After extending the punctum with the punctum dilator and spring scissors and inserting the 0.9 mm diameter probe tip and bent type dacryoendoscope (RUIDO Fiberscope, FiberTech Co., Tokyo, Japan) through the punctum, the internal conditions of the lacrimal duct system were evaluated by passing saline through the upper and lower canaliculus, lacrimal sac, lacrimal duct, and inferior meatus. The obstructive lesion was dislodged by a sheath guided by endoscopy and perfusion solution pressure with a syringe attached to a probe. Under visual guidance, a 0.94 mm-diameter bicanalicular silicone tube (Yoowon Meditec, Seoul, Republic of Korea) was inserted into the sheath. The sheath and tube were retrieved, and both ends of the tube were locked and fixed near the inferior meatus. The tube was removed six months later. According to the clinical course after surgery, levofloxacin 0.5% (cravit®; Santen, Osaka, Japan) and fluorometholone 0.1% (Flumetholone®; Santen, Osaka, Japan) were prescribed.

2.5. Statistical Analysis

SPSS for Windows, version 27.0, was used for all statistical analyses (IBM Corp., Armonk, NY, USA). Parameters were compared using the paired *t*-test, Mann–Whitney test, Kruskal–Wallis test, and Chi-square test. A *p*-value of less than 0.05 was considered statistically significant. Using the Chi-square test, we reported dichotomous outcomes as odds ratios (ORs) and continuous outcomes as the mean and their respective 95% confidence intervals (CIs). Using correlation analysis, the relationships between the categorical variables were examined.

3. Results

There were more women than men in the study (male:female = 8:26). The mean age was 59.50 ± 9.53 years, and the direction of occurrence was comparable. The mean Munk scale was 4.04 ± 1.35, the mean Schirmer test value was 34.77 ± 4.62 mm, and the mean BT was 7.74 ± 2.80 s. The average score on the E-QOL questionnaire was 34.81 ± 17.09 out of 60, the score for daily activity restriction was 13.67 ± 4.50, the score for static activity limit was 13.65 ± 7.58, and the score for dynamic activity limit was 8.92 ± 4.50 (Table 1).

Table 1. Demographics and clinical questionnaires of nasolacrimal duct obstruction (NDO) patients.

	Total (*n* = 34, 48 eyes)
Sex (M:F)	8:26
Age (year)	59.50 ± 9.53
Site (OD:OS)	21:27
Unilateral:Bilateral (n)	20:14
Munk's score	4.04 ± 1.35
Schirmer (mm)	34.77 ± 4.62
BUT (s)	7.74 ± 2.90
E-QOL (60)	34.81 ± 17.09
Daily life restriction (20)	13.67 ± 4.50
Static activity (25)	13.65 ± 7.58
Dynamic activity (15)	8.92 ± 4.65

Comparable to normal, individuals with NDO had a longer CT, and in the case of unilateral NDO, they had a CT that was approximately 60% longer than the opposite eye. After LPI, this reduced similarly to the usual situation. Comparing CT measurements before and after LPI reveals that it reduced by around 60%, leading to an overall decline in BT. After LPI, the TMH had fallen by more than half in all groups. The preoperative CT was longer in the experimental group than in the control group (89.4 ± 20.0 msec versus 140.3 ± 92.0 msec, $p = 0.001$), but there were no other differences. After surgery, the BT (694.4 ± 135.5 msec, 642.4 ± 116.0 msec, $p = 0.032$) and the CT decreased (140.3 ± 92.0 msec, 85.4 ± 22.7 msec, $p < 0.001$), the TMH decreased significantly from 451.5 ± 254.3 µm to 213.7 ± 112.3 µm, the tear film lipid layer thickness remained unchanged, and the BT, CT, CS and OS values were similar to that of the control group (Table 2).

According to the graph of blink dynamics prior to and after surgery, the IPF along the Y-axis fell to 7.61 mm from 8.26 mm. CT reduced from 140.3 msec to 85.4 msec, which is near normal, and BT decreased from 694.4 msec to 642.4 msec, which is also close to normal (Figure 1).

Table 2. Blink pattern and indices of nasolacrimal duct obstruction (NDO) patients before and after lacrimal passage intubation (LPI).

	Normal (48 eyes)	NDO Patients								
		Unilateral (n = 20)			Bilateral (n = 14)			Total (n = 34)		
		Pre	Post	P	Pre	Post	P	Pre	Post	P	Pre	Post	P
Blink pattern										
TB (/20 s)	8.80 ± 5.20	8.32 ± 5.35	9.82 ± 3.55	0.291	8.32 ± 5.35	9.82 ± 3.55	0.252	7.90 ± 4.80	8.29 ± 3.61	0.601	0.224	0.232
PB (/20 s)	4.12 ± 5.62	4.14 ± 3.66	4.25 ± 3.40	0.482	4.14 ± 3.66	4.25 ± 3.40	0.356	3.85 ± 3.96	4.15 ± 3.43	0.561	0.226	0.446
Blink index										
BT (msec)	679.5 ± 98.6	698.3 ± 125.9	650.0 ± 113.2	0.142	691.7 ± 144.2	636.9 ± 119.8	0.086	694.4 ± 135.5	642.4 ± 116.0	0.022	0.715	0.103
LCT (msec)	134.8 ± 35.2	128.3 ± 34.7	125.0 ± 38.9	0.725	136.9 ± 50.0	129.8 ± 26.2	0.433	133.3 ± 44.0	127.8 ± 31.8	0.394	0.746	0.314
CT (msec)	89.4 ± 20.0	140.0 ± 97.1	86.7 ± 16.8	**0.017**	140.5 ± 90.0	84.5 ± 26.4	**0.001**	140.3 ± 92.0	85.4 ± 22.7	**<0.001**	**0.001**	0.377
LOT (msec)	455.3 ± 81.9	430.0 ± 86.5	438.3 ± 99.9	0.770	414.3 ± 85.3	422.6 ± 105.8	0.696	420.8 ± 85.2	429.2 ± 102.6	0.662	0.053	0.183
IBT (msec)	14,563.6 ± 789.0	14,835.0 ± 2772.9	15,993.3 ± 1599.9	0.129	14,164.3 ± 4295.1	13,592.9 ± 3244.0	0.437	14,459.7 ± 3729.7	14,593.1 ± 2917.3	0.779	0.190	0.947
CS (mm/s)	68.54 ± 18.92	69.45 ± 15.90	68.68 ± 24.15	0.873	63.84 ± 17.46	58.96 ± 15.72	0.137	66.18 ± 16.89	63.01 ± 20.03	0.246	0.737	0.178
OS (mm/s)	19.65 ± 3.93	20.39 ± 4.13	19.08 ± 5.81	0.310	20.65 ± 6.58	18.58 ± 5.83	0.060	20.54 ± 5.64	18.79 ± 5.77	0.117	0.511	0.410
IPF (mm)	8.74 ± 1.33	8.51 ± 1.16	7.92 ± 1.17	**0.022**	8.09 ± 1.26	7.39 ± 1.43	**0.002**	8.26 ± 1.23	7.61 ± 1.34	**0.015**	0.052	**0.001**
CT/BT (%)	13.16	20.05	13.34		20.31	13.27		20.20	13.29			
TMH (μm)	-	500.25 ± 232.93	202.20 ± 94.38	**<0.001**	416.61 ± 267.22	221.89 ± 124.60	**<0.001**	451.46 ± 254.34	213.69 ± 112.32	**<0.001**	-	-

NDO, nasolacrimal duct obstruction; TB, total blink; PB, partial blink; BT, blink time; LCT, lid closing time; CT, closure time; LOT, lid opening time; IBT, interblink time; IPF, interpalpebral fissure; CS, closing speed; OS, opening speed. Bold: $p < 0.05$.

The normal control group had a CT during BT ratio of 13.3%, while patients with NDO had a ratio of 19%. After surgery, the CT during BT ratio returned to normal levels (Figure 2A). Before and after surgery, both unilateral and bilateral patients had the same difference, and it can be seen that they have returned to normal after surgery; therefore, the CT during BT is significant (Figure 2B,C). Interestingly, as reported by Su et al. in the 2018 dry eye blink research, CT was also extended in dry eye disease [10]. Secondary epiphora due to dry eye disease similarly lengthened the CT, but when assessed by the ratio in the blink time, it was 7.3% in dry eye patients and 19.1% in patients with NDO, allowing the distinction between the two groups.

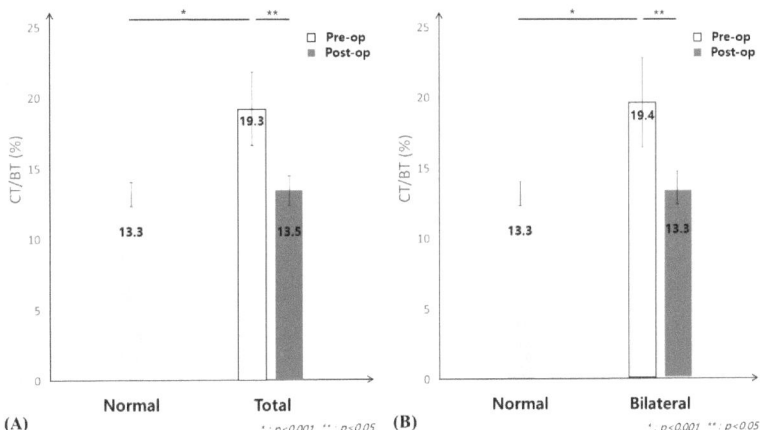

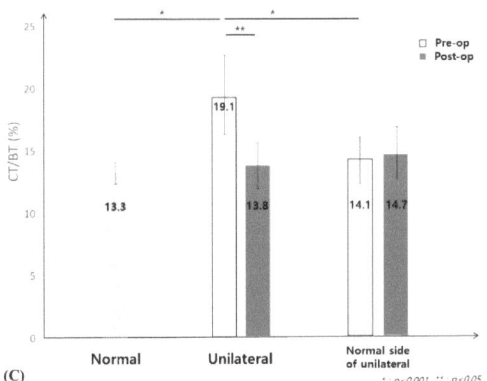

Figure 2. The ratio of index CT during BT (CT/BT) (%) in nasolacrimal duct obstruction (NDO) patients between (**A**) Normal and total NDO patients (**B**) Normal and bilateral NDO patients (**C**) Normal and unilateral NDO patients and the normal side of unilateral NDO patients.

Via an ocular surface-reflecting blink movement study, we sought to identify new indicators that can simultaneously reflect subjective and objective indicators. The blink parameters associated with subjective indicators were BT, CT, and CT during BT; the longer BT and CT were, the greater the ratio of CT during BT, and the stronger the correlation between the E-QOL questionnaire and the objective blink parameters. Objective criteria TMH and punctual reserve showed a positive correlation with the E-QOL questionnaire (Figure 3).

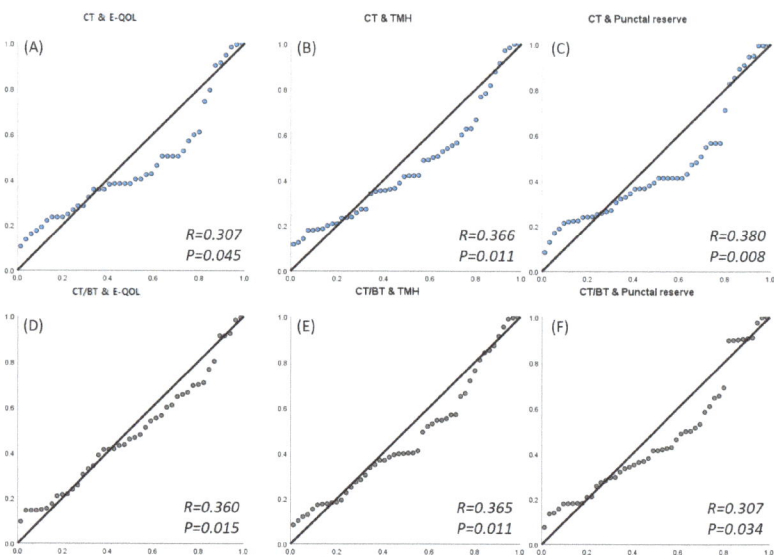

Figure 3. Correlation analysis of the blink index, CT and CT during BT (CT/BT), Quality of Life in Epiphora patients (E-QOL) questionnaire score, tear meniscus height (TMH) and punctal reserve. There are positive correlations with CT and (**A**) Quality of Life in Epiphora patients (E-QOL) questionnaire score, (**B**) tear meniscus height (TMH) and (**C**) punctal reserve. CT during BT (CT/BT) have also positive correlations with CT and (**D**) Quality of Life in Epiphora patients (E-QOL) questionnaire score, (**E**) tear meniscus height (TMH) and (**F**) punctal reserve.

4. Discussion

Several attempts have been undertaken to objectively quantify the quantity of tears shed by individuals who complain of various tear symptoms. TMH, punctal diameter and PR are used to objectively measure the number of stagnant tears [1] as well as the irrigation test, dacryocystography, and dacryoendoscopy, which are used to figure out the precise etiology of NDO. A blink accurately reflects the ocular surface and is associated with the stability of the tear film and the health of the ocular surface [4]. Tse et al. tried to evaluate the clinical–anatomical assessment of NDO patients, including blink dynamics. They suggest the BLICK mnemonic as a useful adjunct to the workup of epiphora (Blink dynamics, Lid malposition, Imbrication, Conjunctivochalasis, and Kissing puncta) [11]. Here, we mainly focus on eyelid blinking in NDO patients because it is believed that the discomfort of retained tears has an effect on eyelid blinking.

The authors' blink profile analysis revealed that NDO patients had a much longer CT and CT during BT than normal controls, and even if only one eye had NDO, the other eye's indices were significantly longer, too. In other words, the eyes were closed for an extended period of time due to greater tear retention caused by NDO, and it returned to normal after LPI. The TMH had decreased after LPI, and the patient's CT and CT during BT normalized after surgery. During eyelid closure or opening, positive/negative pressure spikes are formed throughout the lacrimal duct system, and tears flow via the canaliculus to the lacrimal sac and lacrimal duct, according to Sato et al. [12]. It is believed that longer CT and CT during BT in patients with NDO close eyelids more tightly than usual because tears did not drain under the pressure of normal blinking. They have to squeeze their eyelids to drain the tears. Moreover, CT and CT during BT have demonstrated a positive connection with objective markers (TMH, PR) used to evaluate the absolute amount of tearing in NDO patients (Figure 3, $p < 0.05$). Hence, CT and CT during BT are new measures that can establish the severity of tear retention in patients with NDO.

After LPI, patients' subjective satisfaction may have increased as a result of higher contrast sensitivity, improved vision, decreased blink frequency, and enhanced optical quality [13,14]. Decreased IPF was noted after surgery alongside CT and CT during BT. The exact explanation of this is uncertain; however, it is assumed that the eyes open less due to relative dryness when the LPI-induced tear retention resolves.

For a long time, Munk's scale has been used to measure the level of subjective discomfort. Unfortunately, the Munk scale now in use only represents the number of tears wiped away on a scale of 0 to 5 points, making it difficult to depict the level of discomfort caused by tears in the patient's everyday life. More recently, the TEARS scale and WE-QOL questionnaire [2,3] have been developed. However, in clinical settings, there are a surprising variety of cases in which the objective quantity of stagnant tears (e.g., TMH) and the patient's subjective tear-induced symptoms (e.g., subjective satisfaction, decreased vision) are unrelated. For more precise diagnosis, evaluation and proper treatment of NDO patients, parameters that might reflect subjective symptoms and objectively measured tear amount are becoming necessary. Additionally, the WEQOL questionnaire screened for irritated skin due to tears and primarily focused on unpleasant emotions [3]. On the other hand, there is a distinction in that the E-QOL questionnaire distinguished between static and dynamic activities when confirming the discomfort caused by tears during diverse activities with better specificity. The E-QOL questionnaire also showed a positive correlation with objective parameters, TMH and punctual reserve. Additionally, it also has strong correlation with the other objective parameter, CT, CT during BT (Figure 3, $p < 0.05$).

In this study, 33.3% of patients complained of subjective discomfort due to tears, despite their TMH being below 300 μm. Their CT, CT during BT were higher (175.00 msec) than in the normal group (89.4 msec). In addition, among patients with no subjective discomfort, 12.5% of those show a TMH of 300 μm or above. There might be a considerable gap between objective indicators and subjective symptoms of tears, and it is true that there are complicated interactions among the multiple elements. Since TMH is only the summation of tear secretion and excretion, patients suffering from both dry eye disease and NDO could not demonstrate high TMH. Dry eye syndrome is a typical example of a disorder that causes a significant amount of tear evaporation. NDO, combined with this condition, may suggest normal TMH, which may confound the combined NDO for lower TMH than expected in NDO patients with normal tear secretion. This is the reason why we investigate to discover the clinical parameters of subjective discomfort (E-QOL questionnaire) in accordance with objective parameters (TMH, CT, CT during BT).

Therefore, considering that CT and CT during BT demonstrated a favorable connection with the E-QOL questionnaire scores, CT and CT during BT could be considered as a complementary tool to TMH or the E-QOL questionnaire scores of epiphora patients in diagnosis based on this study. Among them, this was strongly associated with dynamic activities, particularly subjective discomfort, and the correlation between the index value and the CT during BT value showing that patients had poorer quality of life due to tears was significant ($p = 0.001$, $R = 0.489$). Unexpectedly, there was no correlation between Munk's scale and the blink index and E-QOL questionnaire score measured by the investigators. Considering that CT and CT during BT have a correlation with subjective symptoms, it is expected that further studies comparing Munk's scale and blink index with the E-QOL questionnaire will be conducted on a larger number of patients. In addition, CT and CT during BT were correlated with TMH and PR but not with the irrigation test, which could indicate the severity of epiphora symptoms. Future applications may include analyzing instantaneous acceleration and electrode signals during blinking and analyzing them in greater detail than 20 s and 600 frames using a method of tracking eyelid blinking by utilizing continuous blink tracking methods (e.g., a wearable blink tracking device) [4].

CT also demonstrated a protracted pattern of secondary tears resulting from dry eye disease; however, CT during BT was distinct from 19.3% in NDO patients and 7.3% in dry eye patients. According to Su et al., patients with dry eye had longer LCT, LOT, CT, PB, and IBT. Hence, patients with dry eyes blink frequently and slowly. In contrast, LCT, LOT,

PB, and IBT did not differ significantly between NDO patients. Hence, it may be noticed that NDO patients close their eyes longer than those with dry eyes, but other blinking parameters remain the same. This allows us to differentiate this from CT that has been prolonged by secondary tears. Furthermore, additional studies with a larger sample size are anticipated to distinguish between NDO and dry eyes, as well as tears caused by eyelid malposition and tears caused by external stimuli. In addition to blepharospasm, facial palsy, and NDO, it is anticipated that 20 s of blinking image analysis will substantiate the blink pattern of other ophthalmic diseases.

5. Conclusions

CT and CT during BT, which are objective parameters that can also be associated with patients' subjective epiphora symptoms, are considered to be useful parameters for evaluating NDO patients in clinical settings.

Author Contributions: Conceptualization, H.L.; methodology, Y.K. and H.L.; software, Y.K.; validation Y.K.; formal analysis Y.K.; investigation, Y.K.; resources, Y.K.; data curation, Y.K.; writing—original draft preparation, Y.K.; writing—review and editing, Y.K. and H.L.; visualization, Y.K.; supervision, H.L.; project administration, H.L. All authors have read and agreed to the published version of the manuscript.

Funding: This research received no external funding.

Institutional Review Board Statement: The study was conducted in accordance with the Declaration of Helsinki, and approved by the Institutional Review Board of Bundang CHA Medical Center (IRB Number: 2018-12-016) for studies involving humans.

Informed Consent Statement: Patient consent was waived because this study reported on the results of an observational study and complied with the STROBE guidelines.

Data Availability Statement: The data presented in this study are available upon request from the corresponding author. The data are not publicly available due to privacy.

Conflicts of Interest: The authors declare no conflict of interest.

References

1. Sung, Y.; Park, J.S.; Lew, H. Measurement of lacrimal punctum using spectralis domain anterior optical coherence tomography. *Acta Ophthalmol.* **2017**, *95*, e619–e624. [CrossRef]
2. Schulz, C.B.; Malhotra, R. The 'tears' score: A tool for grading and monitoring epiphora. *Eur. J. Ophthalmol.* **2022**, *32*, 2108–2115. [CrossRef] [PubMed]
3. Schulz, C.B.; Rainsbury, P.; Hoffman, J.J.; Ah-Kye, L.; Yang, E.; Malhotra, R.; Rogers, S.; Fayers, P.; Fayers, T. The watery eye quality of life (WEQOL) questionnaire: A patient-reported outcome measure for surgically amenable epiphora. *Eye* **2022**, *36*, 1468–1475. [CrossRef]
4. Rodriguez, J.D.; Lane, K.J.; Ousler, I.I.I.G.W.; Angjeli, E.; Smith, L.M.; Abelson, M.B. Blink: Characteristics, Controls, and Relation to Dry Eyes. *Curr. Eye Res.* **2018**, *43*, 52–66. [CrossRef] [PubMed]
5. Jang, J.; Lew, H. Blink index as a response predictor of blepharospasm to botulinum neurotoxin-A treatment. *Brain Behav.* **2021**, *11*, e2374. [CrossRef]
6. Kim, Y.; Lew, H. Modified blink dynamic index predicts activity and severity in patient with facial nerve palsy. *Front. Ophthalmol.* **2022**, *2*, 960593. [CrossRef]
7. Bartlett, J.D.; Keith, M.S.; Sudharshan, L.; Snedecor, S.J. Associations between signs and symptoms of dry eye disease: A systematic review. *Clin. Ophthalmol.* **2015**, *9*, 1719–1730. [CrossRef] [PubMed]
8. Bacher, L.F.; Allen, K.J. Sensitivity of the rate of spontaneous eye blinking to type of stimuli in young infants. *Dev. Psychobiol.* **2008**, *51*, 186–197. [CrossRef] [PubMed]
9. Lee, S.M.; Lew, H. Transcanalicular endoscopic dacryoplasty in patients with primary acquired nasolacrimal duct obstruction. *Graefe's Arch. Clin. Exp. Ophthalmol.* **2021**, *259*, 173–180. [CrossRef] [PubMed]
10. Su, Y.; Liang, Q.; Su, G.; Wang, N.; Baudouin, C.; Labbé, A. Spontaneous Eye Blink Patterns in Dry Eye: Clinical Correlations. *Investig. Ophthalmol. Vis. Sci.* **2018**, *59*, 5149–5156. [CrossRef] [PubMed]
11. David, T.T.; Erickson, B.P.; Brian, C.T. The BLICK mnemonic for clinical-anatomical assessment of patients with epiphora. *Ophthalmic Plast. Reconstr. Surg.* **2014**, *30*, 450–458.
12. Sato, Y.; Mimura, M.; Fujita, Y.; Oku, H.; Ikeda, T. Chronologic Analysis of Tear Dynamics on Blinking Using Quantitative Manometry in Healthy Humans. *Ophthalmic Plast. Reconstr. Surg.* **2021**, *38*, 22–28. [CrossRef] [PubMed]

13. Hoshi, S.; Tasaki, K.; Hiraoka, T.; Oshika, T. Improvement in Contrast Sensitivity Function after Lacrimal Passage Intubation in Eyes with Epiphora. *J. Clin. Med.* **2020**, *9*, 2761. [CrossRef] [PubMed]
14. Koh, S.; Inoue, Y.; Ochi, S.; Takai, Y.; Maeda, N.; Nishida, K. Quality of Vision in Eyes with Epiphora Undergoing Lacrimal Passage Intubation. *Am. J. Ophthalmol.* **2017**, *181*, 71–78. [CrossRef] [PubMed]

Disclaimer/Publisher's Note: The statements, opinions and data contained in all publications are solely those of the individual author(s) and contributor(s) and not of MDPI and/or the editor(s). MDPI and/or the editor(s) disclaim responsibility for any injury to people or property resulting from any ideas, methods, instructions or products referred to in the content.

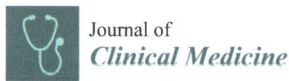

Article

Ocular Surface Changes in Treatment-Naive Thyroid Eye Disease

Xulin Liao [1,†], Kenneth Ka Hei Lai [1,2,†], Fatema Mohamed Ali Abdulla Aljufairi [1,3], Wanxue Chen [1], Zhichao Hu [1], Hanson Yiu Man Wong [1], Ruofan Jia [4], Yingying Wei [4], Clement Chee Yung Tham [1], Chi Pui Pang [1] and Kelvin Kam Lung Chong [1,*]

1. Department of Ophthalmology and Visual Sciences, The Chinese University of Hong Kong, Hong Kong SAR, China
2. Department of Ophthalmology, Tung Wah Eastern Hospital, Hong Kong SAR, China
3. Department of Ophthalmology, Salmaniya Medical Complex, Government Hospitals, Manama 435, Bahrain
4. Department of Statistics, The Chinese University of Hong Kong, Hong Kong SAR, China
* Correspondence: chongkamlung@cuhk.edu.hk; Tel.: +852-3943-5859; Fax: +852-2715-9490
† These authors contributed equally to this work.

Abstract: Objective: To investigate the association of meibomian gland dysfunction (MGD) and ocular surface exposure with tear film instability in untreated thyroid eye disease (TED) patients. Methods: A cross-sectional study of TED patients from September 2020 to September 2022 was conducted. Ocular surface parameters included ocular surface disease index (OSDI), tear meniscus height (TMH), non-invasive tear break-up time (NITBUT), partial blinking rate, lipid layer thickness (LLT), meibomian gland dropout (meiboscore), Schirmer's test, and corneal punctate epithelial erosions (PEE). Ocular surface exposure was assessed by the margin reflex distances of the upper and lower eyelid (MRD1 and MRD2), the amount of exophthalmos, lateral flare, and lagophthalmos. Results: In total, 152 eyes from 76 TED patients (64 females and 12 males, age 42.99 ± 12.28 years) and 93 eyes from 61 healthy controls (51 females and 10 males, age 43.52 ± 17.93 years) were examined. Compared with control eyes, TED eyes had higher OSDI, TMH, LLT, and PEE; shorter NITBUT; and worse meiboscore (all $p < 0.05$). They also had larger amounts of exophthalmos, longer MRD1, more lateral flare, and lagophthalmos. Multivariate analysis identified an association of the tear film instability with lagophthalmos (β = −1.13, 95%CI: −2.08, −0.18) and severe MGD in the lower eyelid (β = −5.01, 95% CI = −7.59, −2.43). Conclusions: Dry eye in TED is mainly manifested as evaporative dry eye disease. Severe lower eyelid MGD and worse lagophthalmos were significantly associated with tear film instability in treatment-naive TED patients.

Keywords: thyroid eye disease; dry eye; meibomian gland dysfunction; non-invasive tear break-up time; lagophthalmos

1. Introduction

Thyroid eye disease (TED), also known as thyroid-associated orbitopathy or Graves ophthalmopathy, is an autoimmune inflammatory disease related to hyperthyroidism or hypothyroidism. However, some TED patients presented as euthyroid [1,2]. TED patients are usually characterized by deformation, diplopia, visual dysfunction, dry eye, and decreased quality of life. The deformation of TED appearance includes exophthalmos, eyelid retraction, eyelid edema, eyelid redness, and lash ptosis [3,4]. The diplopia of TED is related to inflammation or fibrosis of the orbital contents, especially the extraocular muscle [5]. TED threatens vision, especially in dysthyroid optic neuropathy and exposure keratopathy [6]. TED imposes psychological and economic burdens on patients and affects their quality of life [7].

Dry eye symptoms are commonly presented in TED patients [8,9]; some of them have dry eye as the first sign of their ailments. Dry eye disease (DED) is a common eye disease worldwide, affecting around 20% of the population in China [10,11]. According to the Tear Film and Ocular Surface Society Dry Eye Workshop II (TFOS DEWS II) Diagnostic Methodology report, DED can be classified as evaporative and aqueous-deficient dry eye [12]. Evaporative dry eye is characterized by an abnormal lipid layer and is very often caused by meibomian gland dysfunction (MGD). Aqueous deficient dry eye is presented with a low tear meniscus height or Schirmer's test results. The Asia Dry Eye Society (ADES) added decreased wettability caused by the decrease in membrane-associated mucins as a subtype of the DED [13]. DED can be related with or include inflammation, immune dysregulation, lacrimal gland disorders, and MGD [14]. Low-humidity environments, high body mass index, prostaglandin eye drops, and refractive surgery are also risk factors for DED [15,16]. Immune dysregulation and inflammation involving the eyelid, lacrimal gland, and meibomian glands, as well as excessive ocular surface exposure in TED could be risk factors for DED [17]. Moreover, TED treatment by orbital radiation therapy or steroid pulse has been associated with DED [18,19].

This study aims to analyze the meibomian gland dysfunction, ocular surface exposure, and tear film instability in untreated TED patients with a view to appropriately managing these patients at the early stage of their DED.

2. Methods

2.1. Study Design and Subjects

This was a cross-sectional study. The TED patients were recruited from the Chinese University of Hong Kong Medical Centre and the Chinese University of Hong Kong Eye Centre from September 2020 to September 2022. This study adhered to the tenets of the Declaration of Helsinki and Ethics approvals (KC/KE-10-0218/ER-3, NTEC Ref. 2010.594) obtained from the Chinese University of Hong Kong. Inclusion criteria included clinical diagnosis of TED [20]. Patients had to be at least 18 years old and had not received treatment for TED, such as orbital radiation therapy or steroid pulse. Patients with incomplete clinical data, history of refractive or other ocular surgery, ocular trauma, and Sjogren's syndrome were excluded. The healthy controls were age- and sex-matched with the patients, at least 18 years old, and had no underlying ophthalmic diseases. Those who had incomplete clinical data, undergone ophthalmic surgery, or other systemic diseases were excluded.

2.2. Mechanical Ocular Exposure

The margin reflex distance to the upper eyelid (MRD1) is the distance between the upper eyelid margin and the center of the pupillary light reflex in the primary position. The margin reflex distance to the lower eyelid (MRD2) is the distance between the lower eyelid margin to the center of the pupillary light reflex [21]. Exophthalmos was measured by a Hertel exophthalmometer (Keeler Instruments Inc., Broomall, PA, USA). Lagophthalmos is the distance from the upper eyelid margin to the lower eyelid margin when patients close their eyes. Lateral flare is the distance between the upper to lower eyelids just on the lateral side of the corneal limbus [22]. All examinations were conducted by a single senior oculoplastic sub-specialist.

2.3. Dry Eye Assessment

We used the ocular surface disease index (OSDI), which has 12 items and a full score of 100. An OSDI greater than or equal to 13 was regarded as subjective dry eye [23]. The average, maximum, and minimum lipid layer thickness (av-LLT, max-LLT, min-LLT, respectively) and meibography were measured using a Lipiview interferometer (TearScience Inc., Morrisville, NC, USA) [24]. The grading scheme of meibography is the meiboscore (0–3 score for one eyelid) [25]. We regarded 0 and 1 as mild, 2 as moderate, and 3 as severe meibomian gland dysfunction. The tear meniscus height (TMH) and first and average non-invasive tear break-up time (f-NITBUT, av-NITBUT, respectively) were measured by an OCULUS keratograph 5M (Oculus Optikgerate, Wetzer, Germany) [26]. Schirmer's test (ST-I) without anesthesia was used to test the aqueous tear production. Ocular surface fluorescein staining under a slit lamp was used to evaluate the punctate epithelial erosions (PEE). We applied the Oxford grading scheme (0–6 score) to evaluate the severity of PEE [27].

2.4. Statistical Analysis

The continuous variables were presented as mean ± standard deviation. The binary variables were expressed as percentages. The two-group comparison used the Student *t*-test for continuous variables and the Chi-square test for categorical variables. We also conducted univariate and multivariate linear regression to estimate the association of orbital and ocular surface parameters and TED. For the multivariate linear regression model, we adjusted the cofounder, including age, sex, and smoking status. The generalized estimating equation was used to adjust the inter-correlation between two eyes from the same subject. 3 Linear regression models were employed to examine the difference between TED and healthy controls by using orbital and ocular surface parameters as dependent variables. We also applied linear regression models to identify the relationship between the first NITBUT, orbital and ocular surface parameters by utilizing the first NITBUT as the dependent variable. A *p* value less than 0.05 was considered statistically significant. All the statistical analyses were performed using SPSS (IBM SPSS 23.0, SPSS Inc. Armonk, NY, USA) and R-Software R Project https://www.r-project.org/ accessed on 9 March 2023.

3. Results

3.1. Demographic and Clinical Features of TED Patients and Healthy Controls

We recruited 76 TED patients (152 eyes) and 61 healthy controls (93 eyes) who were age and sex matched (Table 1) Among them, 19.74% TED patients were smokers versus 4.92% of controls. Additionally, 72.37% of TED patients had Graves' disease. Compared to the controls, the TED patients had larger amounts of exophthalmos, longer MRD1, larger lateral flare, and greater lagophthalmos with statistical significance (Table 2). For the dry eye parameters, the TED patients had higher OSDI, increased TMH, shorter f-NITBUT, shorter av-NITBUT, higher av-LLT, worse meiboscore in both the upper eyelid and lower eyelid, and more severe PEE than the controls with significant differences.

Table 1. Demographics characteristics of thyroid eye disease (TED) and healthy controls.

	TED	Healthy Controls	*p*-Value
Subject numbers	76	61	
Age (years)	42.99 ± 12.28	43.52 ± 17.93	0.836
Onset age (years)	41.26 ± 13.17	NA	
Female:Male	64:12	51:10	0.924
Clinical activity score	0.88 ± 1.19	NA	
Graves' disease (N%) [#]	55 (72.37%)	0 (0.00%)	<0.001
Smoker (N%) [#]	15 (19.74%)	3 (4.92%)	0.011

[#] Chi-square test.

Table 2. Clinical characteristics of thyroid eye disease (TED) and healthy controls.

	TED	Healthy Controls	*p*-Value
Eye numbers	152	93	
Visual acuity (Log MAR)	0.97 ± 0.16	1.09 ± 0.30	<0.001
Orbital parameters			
Exophthalmos (mm)	18.09 ± 2.95	16.29 ± 1.59	<0.001
MRD1 (mm)	5.36 ± 1.63	4.03 ± 0.90	<0.001
MRD2 (mm)	5.03 ± 0.98	5.04 ± 0.55	0.638
Lateral flare (mm)	9.74 ± 2.20	7.23 ± 1.58	<0.001
Lagophthalmos (mm)	0.55 ± 0.88	0.00 ± 0.00	<0.001
Ocular surface parameters			
OSDI	28.01 ± 21.70	5.64 ± 3.59	<0.001

Table 2. Cont.

	TED	Healthy Controls	p-Value
Schirmer's test (mm)	13.67 ± 10.22	12.97 ± 9.57	0.593
TMH (mm)	0.33 ± 0.17	0.26 ± 0.11	<0.001
f-NITBUT (s)	10.16 ± 5.96	15.40 ± 3.71	<0.001
av-NITBUT (s)	15.58 ± 4.71	17.53 ± 2.91	<0.001
av-LLT (nm)	71.03 ± 23.41	62.99 ± 20.53	0.007
max-LLT (nm)	84.84 ± 19.42	79.99 ± 18.74	0.056
min-LLT (nm)	54.64 ± 23.47	50.57 ± 18.92	0.159
Meiboscore upper eyelid	1.64 ± 0.85	1.34 ± 0.63	0.004
Meiboscore lower eyelid	1.36 ± 0.65	1.12 ± 0.69	0.006
Punctate epithelial erosions	0.85 ± 0.73	0.27 ± 0.47	<0.001

Abbreviations: MRD1, margin reflex distance of the upper eyelid; MRD2, margin reflex distance of the lower eyelid; OSDI, ocular surface disease index; TMH, tear meniscus height; f-NITBUT, first non-invasive tear break up time; av-NITBUT, average non-invasive tear break up time; av-LLT, average lipid layer thickness; max-LLT, maximum lipid layer thickness; min-LLT, minimum lipid layer thickness.

3.2. Association of Orbital and Ocular Surface Parameters in TED and Healthy Controls

As shown in Table 3, after adjusting the confounders, including age, sex, and smoking status, the multivariate model showed that TED was associated with exophthalmos, MRD1, lateral flare, lagophthalmos, OSDI, TMH, f-NITBUT, av-NIKBUT, av-LLT, meiboscore in the upper eyelid, meiboscore in the lower eyelid, and PEE. Therefore, the TED patients had more ocular surface exposure, severe objective dry eye symptoms, more unstable tear film, reflex tearing, increased lipid layer thickness, worse evaporative dry eye, and more PEE (Tables 2 and 3) than healthy controls. Thus, they mainly manifested as having evaporative dry eyes rather than aqueous deficient dry eyes.

Table 3. Association of orbital and ocular surface parameters in thyroid eye disease and healthy controls (245 eyes).

	Univariate Model			Multivariate Model *		
	β	95%CI	p-Value	β	95%CI	p-Value
Orbital parameters						
Exophthalmos (mm)	1.80	1.03, 2.57	<0.001	1.77	0.96, 2.59	<0.001
MRD1 (mm)	1.32	0.94, 1.71	<0.001	1.25	0.85, 1.65	<0.001
MRD2 (mm)	−0.01	−0.25, 0.23	0.933	−0.04	−0.28, 0.21	0.768
Lateral flare (mm)	2.52	1.92, 3.12	<0.001	2.55	1.96, 3.14	<0.001
Lagophthalmos (mm)	0.55	0.36, 0.73	<0.001	0.61	0.40, 0.81	<0.001
Ocular surface parameters						
OSDI	22.38	17.39, 27.36	<0.001	20.93	16.10, 25.76	<0.001
Schirmer's test (mm)	0.70	−2.53, 3.94	0.670	0.62	−2.68, 3.91	0.713
TMH (mm)	0.07	0.03, 0.11	0.002	0.07	0.02, 0.12	0.003
f−NITBUT (s)	−5.24	−6.54, −3.94	<0.001	−5.13	−6.51, −3.74	<0.001
av-NITBUT (s)	−1.94	−3.06, −0.83	0.001	−1.84	−2.97, −0.70	0.002
av-LLT (nm)	8.04	1.14, 14.93	0.022	8.99	1.90, 16.09	0.013
max-LLT (nm)	4.85	−1.13, 10.83	0.112	5.56	−0.56, 11.68	0.075
min-LLT (nm)	4.07	−2.44, 10.58	0.221	5.62	−1.12, 12.37	0.102
Meiboscore upper eyelid	0.29	0.05, 0.54	0.017	0.30	0.05, 0.55	0.017
Meiboscore lower eyelid	0.24	0.04, 0.45	0.018	0.21	0.01, 0.42	0.040
Punctate epithelial erosions	0.58	0.40, 0.76	<0.001	0.55	0.37, 0.73	<0.001

* Adjust: Age, Sex, Smoker. Abbreviations: MRD1, margin reflex distance of the upper eyelid; MRD2, margin reflex distance of the lower eyelid; OSDI, ocular surface disease index; TMH, tear meniscus height; f-NITBUT, first non-invasive tear break up time; av-NITBUT, average non-invasive tear break up time; av-LLT, average lipid layer thickness; max-LLT, maximum lipid layer thickness; min-LLT, minimum lipid layer thickness.

3.3. Association of Tear Film Instability (f-NITBUT) and Clinical Parameters in TED and Healthy Controls

Tear film instability was associated with the lagophthalmos and severe MGD in the lower eyelid (Table 4). After controlling other factors, for every 1 mm increase in lagophthalmos in TED patients, the non-invasive tear break-up time was shortened by 1.13 s. In comparison to mild MGD in the lower eyelid, the tear break-up time in severe

MGD was reduced by 5.01 s. However, the control group did not show any association between the clinical parameters and tear film instability (Table 5).

Table 4. Association of tear film instability and clinical parameters in thyroid eye disease (152 eyes).

	Univariate Model			Multivariate Model *		
	β	95%CI	p-Value	β	95%CI	p-Value
Orbit parameters						
Exophthalmos (mm)	0.10	−0.29, 0.50	0.602	−0.02	−0.37, 0.32	0.898
MRD1 (mm)	−0.33	−0.97, 0.31	0.310	−0.36	−0.96, 0.24	0.243
MRD2 (mm)	0.71	−0.27, 1.69	0.157	0.63	−0.32, 1.57	0.192
Lateral flare (mm)	−0.15	−0.66, 0.35	0.545	−0.25	−0.70, 0.21	0.292
Lagophthalmos (mm)	−0.82	−1.66, 0.03	0.060	−1.13	−2.08, −0.18	0.020
Ocular surface parameters						
Schirmer's test (mm)	−0.01	−0.10, 0.09	0.874	−0.03	−0.12, 0.06	0.490
TMH (mm)	2.55	−3.55, 8.64	0.413	1.25	−4.21, 6.70	0.654
av-LLT (nm)	−0.02	−0.05, 0.02	0.336	−0.01	−0.04, 0.03	0.732
max-LLT (nm)	0.00	−0.04, 0.04	0.840	0.02	−0.03, 0.06	0.451
min-LLT (nm)	−0.02	−0.06, 0.02	0.350	−0.02	−0.05, 0.02	0.400
Punctate epithelial erosions	−1.30	−2.45, −0.16	0.026	−1.08	−2.21, 0.05	0.061
Meiboscore upper eyelid						
Mild	Reference			Reference		
Moderate	0.49	−1.81, 2.79	0.678	1.15	−1.11, 3.40	0.318
Severe	−0.33	−3.40, 2.73	0.830	−0.28	−3.06, 2.50	0.842
Meiboscore lower eyelid						
Mild	Reference			Reference		
Moderate	0.82	−1.56, 3.20	0.498	0.83	−1.36, 3.02	0.459
Severe	−5.21	−7.74, −2.68	<0.001	−5.01	−7.59, −2.43	<0.001

* Adjust: Age, Sex, Smoker. Abbreviations: MRD1, margin reflex distance of the upper eyelid; MRD2, margin reflex distance of the lower eyelid; OSDI, ocular surface disease index; TMH, tear meniscus height; av-NITBUT, average non-invasive tear break up time; av-LLT, average lipid layer thickness; max-LLT, maximum lipid layer thickness; min-LLT, minimum lipid layer thickness.

Table 5. Association of tear film instability and clinical parameters in healthy controls (93 eyes).

	Univariate Model			Multivariate Model *		
	β	95%CI	p-Value	β	95%CI	p-Value
Orbit parameters						
Exophthalmos (mm)	−0.01	−0.45, 0.43	0.968	−0.01	−0.46, 0.44	0.962
MRD1 (mm)	0.37	−0.44, 1.18	0.371	0.39	−0.47, 1.24	0.378
MRD2 (mm)	0.67	−0.95, 2.29	0.420	0.67	−0.95, 2.28	0.419
Lateral flare (mm)	0.03	−0.39, 0.45	0.891	0.04	−0.38, 0.46	0.853
Ocular surface parameters						
Schirmer's test (mm)	−0.01	−0.09, 0.08	0.831	−0.01	−0.10, 0.08	0.839
TMH (mm)	−1.79	−8.98, 5.41	0.626	−2.13	−9.40, 5.14	0.567
av-LLT (nm)	−0.02	−0.05, 0.02	0.368	−0.02	−0.06, 0.02	0.336
max-LLT (nm)	−0.02	−0.06, 0.02	0.271	−0.02	−0.06, 0.02	0.259
min-LLT (nm)	0.00	−0.04, 0.04	0.943	0.00	−0.04, 0.04	0.970
Punctate epithelial erosions	−0.76	−2.26, 0.74	0.319	−0.82	−2.48, 0.84	0.335
Meiboscore upper eyelid						
Mild	Reference			Reference		
Moderate	−0.67	−2.50, 1.17	0.476	−1.01	−3.05, 1.03	0.334
Severe	−0.56	−1.99, 0.87	0.443	−0.65	−1.91, 0.61	0.310
Meiboscore lower eyelid						
Mild	Reference			Reference		
Moderate	0.26	−2.11, 2.63	0.831	0.30	−2.55, 3.15	0.838
Severe	0.30	−4.15, 4.74	0.896	0.17	−4.39, 4.72	0.943

* Adjust: Age, Sex, Smoker. Abbreviations: MRD1, margin reflex distance of the upper eyelid; MRD2, margin reflex distance of the lower eyelid; OSDI, ocular surface disease index; TMH, tear meniscus height; av-NITBUT, average non-invasive tear break up time; av-LLT, average lipid layer thickness; max-LLT, maximum lipid layer thickness; min-LLT, minimum lipid layer thickness.

4. Discussion

In this cross-sectional study, we found an association of lower eyelid meibomian gland dropout and lagophthalmos with tear film instability in untreated TED. MGD has a significant impact on the dry eye status of untreated TED patients. Our study found that the influence of MGD on tear film instability is even greater than the impact of mechanical exposure factors.

Treatment-naïve TED patients mainly manifested as having evaporative dry eyes rather than aqueous deficient dry eyes. Many studies have shown that TED patients will have worsened MGD, as Kim et al. reported that TED patients have a higher prevalence of obstructive type MGD [28], and Tugan reported that the meibomian glands are quantitatively decreased in patients with TED [29]. In this study we further proved that the evaporative dry eye rather than the aqueous deficient dry eye affects untreated TED dry eye symptoms. Some studies mentioned that radiation therapy would affect meibomian glands [18] and worsen dry eye [30]. However, other studies reported improvement of the MGD [31] after treatment by steroid pulse and orbital radiation therapies in active thyroid eye disease.

The tear meniscus height in TED patients was higher than in healthy controls in this study. Both TMH and ST were greater than in healthy controls. A TMH of more than 0.25 mm could indicate that reflex tearing had been reported [32], likely due to the exposure of the eyeball that stimulates the lacrimal glands to secrete tears [33,34]. In some TED patients, the inflammation and swelling could affect the lacrimal gland and disrupt its ability to produce tears [35]. Thus, the relationship between the lacrimal gland and dry eye parameters in TED patients need further investigation.

The MGD in the lower eyelid affects tear film instability in untreated TED. Based on the results of this and other studies, both the upper and lower eyelid meibomian glands are likely to be impaired in TED [36,37]. However, severe deficiency of the lower eyelid meibomian gland significantly impacts tear film stability in TED compared to the upper eyelid MGD. We speculate that this is because the upper eyelid occupies a greater volume and area than the lower eyelid. Thyroid eye disease can cause enlargement of the extraocular muscles or fat, resulting in an increase in the contents of the eye. As a result, when the patient blinks their eyes, a large area of the upper eyelid is squeezed. Therefore, the meibomian gland function of the upper eyelid is slightly better than that of the lower eyelid [38]. Blinking with pressure assists the obstructive meibomian gland to have better secretion. According to the findings of this study, we would recommend gentle compressions and massage during the early stage of TED to produce more relief, especially for the lower eyelid. We also found greater lipid layer thickness in TED than in controls, consistent with reported patients of active TED having more severe MGD but thicker LLT [39]. We think that the TED MGD might be seborrheic MGD [40], with excessive secretion of cloudy meibomian lipids. Moreover, the inflammation of eye contents also affects the meibomian gland and the poor secretion quality of the meibum [41]. Lagophthalmos is incomplete eyelid closure, which results in exposure keratitis [42,43]. Therefore, wearing an eye patch for lagophthalmos during sleep may be beneficial for relieving dry eye symptoms in patients with TED.

Results of this study revealed the relationship between tear film instability, ocular surface exposure, MGD, and other dry eye parameters in untreated TED. There should be attention paid to manage MGD at an early stage in TED. However, this study had the limitation of not evaluating the blinking mechanism and biophysical properties of meibum, which may affect the dry eye status in TED.

In conclusion, treatment-naive TED patients have poor ocular surface status both in objective and subjective dry eye parameters, which mainly manifested as evaporative dry eyes. Lower eyelid MGD and worse lagophthalmos were significantly associated with tear film instability in treatment-naive TED patients. For untreated TED patients, the dry eye status should not be ignored, and the management approach should mainly focus on meibomian gland dysfunction and lagophthalmos.

Author Contributions: Conceptualization, C.C.Y.T. and C.P.P.; Methodology, W.C., Z.H. and H.Y.M.W.; Software, W.C., Z.H. and H.Y.M.W.; Validation, K.K.L.C.; Formal analysis, X.L., R.J. and Y.W.; Investigation, K.K.H.L. and F.M.A.A.A.; Resources, C.C.Y.T. and C.P.P.; Data curation, X.L., R.J. and Y.W.; Writing—original draft, X.L.; Writing—review & editing, K.K.H.L., F.M.A.A.A., C.C.Y.T., C.P.P.

and K.K.L.C.; Supervision, K.K.L.C.; Project administration, C.C.Y.T. and C.P.P. All authors have read and agreed to the published version of the manuscript.

Funding: This research received no external funding.

Institutional Review Board Statement: The study was conducted in accordance with the Declaration of Helsinki, and approved by the Joint CUHK-NTEC Clinical Research Ethics Committee (protocol code KC/KE-10-0218/ER-3, NTEC Ref. 2010.594 and date of approval 20 January 2011).

Informed Consent Statement: Informed consent was obtained from all subjects involved in the study.

Data Availability Statement: Not applicable.

Conflicts of Interest: The authors declare no conflict of interest.

References

1. Bartalena, L.; Kahaly, G.J.; Baldeschi, L.; Dayan, C.M.; Eckstein, A.; Marcocci, C.; Marinò, M.; Vaidya, B.; Wiersinga, W.M.; EUGOGO. The 2021 European Group on Graves' orbitopathy (EUGOGO) clinical practice guidelines for the medical management of Graves' orbitopathy. *Eur. J. Endocrinol.* **2021**, *185*, G43–G67. [CrossRef]
2. Boulakh, L.; Nygaard, B.; Bek, T.; Faber, J.; Heegaard, S.; Toft, P.B.; Poulsen, H.E.; Toft-Petersen, A.P.; Hesgaard, H.B.; Ellervik, C. Nationwide Incidence of Thyroid Eye Disease and Cumulative Incidence of Strabismus and Surgical Interventions in Denmark. *JAMA Ophthalmol.* **2022**, *140*, 667–673. [CrossRef]
3. Duan, M.; Xu, D.D.; Zhou, H.L.; Fang, H.Y.; Meng, W.; Wang, Y.N.; Jin, Z.Y.; Chen, Y.; Zhang, Z.H. Triamcinolone acetonide injection in the treatment of upper eyelid retraction in Graves' ophthalmopathy evaluated by 3.0 Tesla magnetic resonance imaging. *Indian J. Ophthalmol.* **2022**, *70*, 1736–1741. [PubMed]
4. Yu, C.Y.; Ford, R.L.; Wester, S.T.; Shriver, E.M. Update on thyroid eye disease: Regional variations in prevalence, diagnosis, and management. *Indian J. Ophthalmol.* **2022**, *70*, 2335–2345. [PubMed]
5. Kahaly, G.J.; Douglas, R.S.; Holt, R.J.; Sile, S.; Smith, T.J. Teprotumumab for patients with active thyroid eye disease: A pooled data analysis, subgroup analyses, and off-treatment follow-up results from two randomised, double-masked, placebo-controlled, multicentre trials. *Lancet Diabetes Endocrinol.* **2021**, *9*, 360–372. [CrossRef] [PubMed]
6. Wu, H.; Luo, B.; Wang, Q.; Zhao, Y.; Yuan, G.; Liu, P.; Zhai, L.; Lv, W.; Zhang, J. Functional and Morphological Brain Alterations in Dysthyroid Optic Neuropathy: A Combined Resting-State fMRI and Voxel-Based Morphometry Study. *J. Magn. Reson. Imaging JMRI* **2022**. [CrossRef]
7. Sharma, A.; Stan, M.N.; Rootman, D.B. Measuring Health-Related Quality of Life in Thyroid Eye Disease. *J. Clin. Endocrinol. Metab.* **2022**, *107*, S27–S35. [CrossRef]
8. Carreira, A.R.; Rodrigues-Barros, S.; Moraes, F.; Loureiro, T.; Machado, I.; Campos, P.; Nobre Cardoso, J.; Campos, N. Impact of Graves Disease on Ocular Surface and Corneal Epithelial Thickness in Patients with and without Graves Orbitopathy. *Cornea* **2022**, *41*, 443–449. [CrossRef]
9. Gürdal, C.; Saraç, O.; Genç, I.; Kırımlıoğlu, H.; Takmaz, T.; Can, I. Ocular surface and dry eye in Graves' disease. *Curr. Eye Res.* **2011**, *36*, 8–13. [CrossRef]
10. Jie, Y.; Xu, L.; Wu, Y.Y.; Jonas, J.B. Prevalence of dry eye among adult Chinese in the Beijing Eye Study. *Eye* **2009**, *23*, 688–693. [CrossRef]
11. Craig, J.P.; Nichols, K.K.; Akpek, E.K.; Caffery, B.; Dua, H.S.; Joo, C.K.; Liu, Z.; Nelson, J.D.; Nichols, J.J.; Tsubota, K.; et al. TFOS DEWS II Definition and Classification Report. *Ocul. Surf.* **2017**, *15*, 276–283. [CrossRef] [PubMed]
12. Wolffsohn, J.S.; Arita, R.; Chalmers, R.; Djalilian, A.; Dogru, M.; Dumbleton, K.; Gupta, P.K.; Karpecki, P.; Lazreg, S.; Pult, H.; et al. TFOS DEWS II Diagnostic Methodology report. *Ocul. Surf.* **2017**, *15*, 539–574. [CrossRef]
13. Tsubota, K.; Yokoi, N.; Shimazaki, J.; Watanabe, H.; Dogru, M.; Yamada, M.; Kinoshita, S.; Kim, H.M.; Tchah, H.W.; Hyon, J.Y.; et al. New Perspectives on Dry Eye Definition and Diagnosis: A Consensus Report by the Asia Dry Eye Society. *Ocul. Surf.* **2017**, *15*, 65–76. [CrossRef] [PubMed]
14. Kojima, T.; Dogru, M.; Kawashima, M.; Nakamura, S.; Tsubota, K. Advances in the diagnosis and treatment of dry eye. *Prog. Retin. Eye Res.* **2020**, *78*, 100842. [CrossRef]
15. Netto, A.R.T.; Hurst, J.; Bartz-Schmidt, K.U.; Schnichels, S. Porcine Corneas Incubated at Low Humidity Present Characteristic Features Found in Dry Eye Disease. *Int. J. Mol. Sci.* **2022**, *23*, 4567. [CrossRef] [PubMed]
16. Alkhaldi, S.A.; Allam, K.H.; Radwan, M.A.; Sweeny, L.E.; Alshammeri, S. Estimates of dry eye disease in Saudi Arabia based on a short questionnaire of prevalence, symptoms, and risk factors: The Twaiq Mountain Eye Study I. *Contact Lens Anterior Eye J. Br. Contact Lens Assoc.* **2022**, *46*, 101770. [CrossRef]
17. Rana, H.S.; Akella, S.S.; Clabeaux, C.E.; Skurski, Z.P.; Aakalu, V.K. Ocular surface disease in thyroid eye disease: A narrative review. *Ocul. Surf.* **2022**, *24*, 67–73. [CrossRef]
18. Kim, S.E.; Yang, H.J.; Yang, S.W. Effects of radiation therapy on the meibomian glands and dry eye in patients with ocular adnexal mucosa-associated lymphoid tissue lymphoma. *BMC Ophthalmol.* **2020**, *20*, 24. [CrossRef]

19. Sabeti, S.; Kheirkhah, A.; Yin, J.; Dana, R. Management of meibomian gland dysfunction: A review. *Surv. Ophthalmol.* **2020**, *65*, 205–217. [CrossRef]
20. Bartley, G.B.; Gorman, C.A. Diagnostic criteria for Graves' ophthalmopathy. *Am. J. Ophthalmol.* **1995**, *119*, 792–795. [CrossRef]
21. Paik, J.S.; Han, K.; Yang, S.W.; Park, Y.; Na, K.; Cho, W.; Jung, S.K.; Kim, S. Blepharoptosis among Korean adults: Age-related prevalence and threshold age for evaluation. *BMC Ophthalmol.* **2020**, *20*, 99. [CrossRef]
22. Park, H.H.; Chun, Y.S.; Moon, N.J.; Kim, J.T.; Park, S.J.; Lee, J.K. Change in eyelid parameters after orbital decompression in thyroid-associated orbitopathy. *Eye* **2018**, *32*, 1036–1041. [CrossRef]
23. Dougherty, B.E.; Nichols, J.J.; Nichols, K.K. Rasch analysis of the Ocular Surface Disease Index (OSDI). *Investig. Ophthalmol. Vis. Sci.* **2011**, *52*, 8630–8635. [CrossRef] [PubMed]
24. Finis, D.; Pischel, N.; Schrader, S.; Geerling, G. Evaluation of lipid layer thickness measurement of the tear film as a diagnostic tool for Meibomian gland dysfunction. *Cornea* **2013**, *32*, 1549–1553. [CrossRef] [PubMed]
25. Arita, R.; Itoh, K.; Inoue, K.; Amano, S. Noncontact infrared meibography to document age-related changes of the meibomian glands in a normal population. *Ophthalmology* **2008**, *115*, 911–915. [CrossRef]
26. Kolbe, O.; Zimmermann, F.; Marx, S.; Sickenberger, W. Introducing a novel in vivo method to access visual performance during dewetting process of contact lens surface. *Contact Lens Anterior Eye J. Br. Contact Lens Assoc.* **2020**, *43*, 359–365. [CrossRef] [PubMed]
27. Chien, K.J.; Horng, C.T.; Huang, Y.S.; Hsieh, Y.H.; Wang, C.J.; Yang, J.S.; Lu, C.C.; Chen, F.A. Effects of *Lycium barbarum* (goji berry) on dry eye disease in rats. *Mol. Med. Rep.* **2018**, *17*, 809–818. [CrossRef]
28. Kim, Y.S.; Kwak, A.Y.; Lee, S.Y.; Yoon, J.S.; Jang, S.Y. Meibomian gland dysfunction in Graves' orbitopathy. *Can. J. Ophthalmol. J. Can. D'ophtalmologie* **2015**, *50*, 278–282. [CrossRef]
29. Yılmaz Tuğan, B.; Özkan, B. Evaluation of Meibomian Gland Loss and Ocular Surface Changes in Patients with Mild and Moderate-to-Severe Graves' Ophthalmopathy. *Semin. Ophthalmol.* **2022**, *37*, 271–276. [CrossRef] [PubMed]
30. Wang, K.; Tobillo, R.; Mavroidis, P.; Pappafotis, R.; Pearlstein, K.A.; Moon, D.H.; Mahbooba, Z.M.; Deal, A.M.; Holmes, J.A.; Sheets, N.C.; et al. Prospective Assessment of Patient-Reported Dry Eye Syndrome after Whole Brain Radiation. *Int. J. Radiat. Oncol. Biol. Phys.* **2019**, *105*, 765–772. [CrossRef]
31. Takahashi, Y.; Vaidya, A.; Kakizaki, H. Changes in Dry Eye Status after Steroid Pulse and Orbital Radiation Therapies in Active Thyroid Eye Disease. *J. Clin. Med.* **2022**, *11*, 3604. [CrossRef]
32. Doughty, M.J.; Laiquzzaman, M.; Oblak, E.; Button, N. The tear (lacrimal) meniscus height in human eyes: A useful clinical measure or an unusable variable sign? *Contact Lens Anterior Eye J. Br. Contact Lens Assoc.* **2002**, *25*, 57–65. [CrossRef]
33. Wu, Z.; Begley, C.G.; Port, N.; Bradley, A.; Braun, R.; King-Smith, E. The Effects of Increasing Ocular Surface Stimulation on Blinking and Tear Secretion. *Investig. Ophthalmol. Vis. Sci.* **2015**, *56*, 4211–4220. [CrossRef] [PubMed]
34. Wu, Z.; Begley, C.G.; Situ, P.; Simpson, T. The effects of increasing ocular surface stimulation on blinking and sensation. *Investig. Ophthalmol. Vis. Sci.* **2014**, *55*, 1555–1563. [CrossRef] [PubMed]
35. Razek, A.A.; El-Hadidy, E.M.; Moawad, M.E.; El-Metwaly, N.; El-Said, A.A.E. Assessment of lacrimal glands in thyroid eye disease with diffusion-weighted magnetic resonance imaging. *Pol. J. Radiol.* **2019**, *84*, e142–e146. [CrossRef]
36. Inoue, S.; Kawashima, M.; Arita, R.; Kozaki, A.; Tsubota, K. Investigation of Meibomian Gland Function and Dry Eye Disease in Patients with Graves' Ophthalmopathy. *J. Clin. Med.* **2020**, *9*, 2814. [CrossRef] [PubMed]
37. Park, J.; Kim, J.; Lee, H.; Park, M.; Baek, S. Functional and structural evaluation of the meibomian gland using a LipiView interferometer in thyroid eye disease. *Can. J. Ophthalmol. J. Can. D'ophtalmol.* **2018**, *53*, 373–379. [CrossRef] [PubMed]
38. Eom, Y.; Choi, K.E.; Kang, S.Y.; Lee, H.K.; Kim, H.M.; Song, J.S. Comparison of meibomian gland loss and expressed meibum grade between the upper and lower eyelids in patients with obstructive meibomian gland dysfunction. *Cornea* **2014**, *33*, 448–452. [CrossRef]
39. Wang, C.Y.; Ho, R.W.; Fang, P.C.; Yu, H.J.; Chien, C.C.; Hsiao, C.C.; Kuo, M.T. The function and morphology of Meibomian glands in patients with thyroid eye disease: A preliminary study. *BMC Ophthalmol.* **2018**, *18*, 90. [CrossRef]
40. Nelson, J.D.; Shimazaki, J.; Benitez-del-Castillo, J.M.; Craig, J.P.; McCulley, J.P.; Den, S.; Foulks, G.N. The international workshop on meibomian gland dysfunction: Report of the definition and classification subcommittee. *Investig. Ophthalmol. Vis. Sci.* **2011**, *52*, 1930–1937. [CrossRef]
41. Farid, M.; Agrawal, A.; Fremgen, D.; Tao, J.; Chuyi, H.; Nesburn, A.B.; BenMohamed, L. Age-related Defects in Ocular and Nasal Mucosal Immune System and the Immunopathology of Dry Eye Disease. *Ocul. Immunol. Inflamm.* **2016**, *24*, 327–347. [CrossRef] [PubMed]
42. Rita, M.R.H.; Deepa, M.; Gitanjali, V.C.; Tinu, S.R.; Subbulakshmi, B.; Sujitha, D.; Palthya, G.; Saradha, M.; Vedhavalli, T.; Sowmiya, B.; et al. Lagophthalmos: An etiological lookout to frame the decision for management. *Indian J. Ophthalmol.* **2022**, *70*, 3077–3082. [CrossRef] [PubMed]
43. Patel, V.; Daya, S.M.; Lake, D.; Malhotra, R. Blink lagophthalmos and dry eye keratopathy in patients with non-facial palsy: Clinical features and management with upper eyelid loading. *Ophthalmology* **2011**, *118*, 197–202. [CrossRef] [PubMed]

Disclaimer/Publisher's Note: The statements, opinions and data contained in all publications are solely those of the individual author(s) and contributor(s) and not of MDPI and/or the editor(s). MDPI and/or the editor(s) disclaim responsibility for any injury to people or property resulting from any ideas, methods, instructions or products referred to in the content.

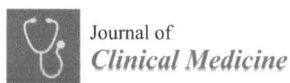 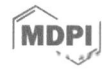

Article

Clinical Significance of Corneal Striae in Thyroid Associated Orbitopathy

Xulin Liao [1], Fatema Mohamed Ali Abdulla Aljufairi [1,2], Kenneth Ka Hei Lai [1,3], Karen Kar Wun Chan [1,4], Ruofan Jia [5], Wanxue Chen [1], Zhichao Hu [1], Yingying Wei [5], Winnie Chiu Wing Chu [6], Clement Chee Yung Tham [1], Chi Pui Pang [1] and Kelvin Kam Lung Chong [1,4,*]

[1] Department of Ophthalmology and Visual Sciences, The Chinese University of Hong Kong, Hong Kong SAR, China
[2] Department of Ophthalmology, Salmaniya Medical Complex, Government Hospitals, Manama 435, Bahrain
[3] Department of Ophthalmology, Tung Wah Eastern Hospital, Hong Kong SAR, China
[4] Department of Ophthalmology and Visual Sciences, Prince of Wales Hospital, Hong Kong SAR, China
[5] Department of Statistics, The Chinese University of Hong Kong, Hong Kong SAR, China
[6] Department of Imaging and Interventional Radiology, Faculty of Medicine, The Prince of Wales Hospital, The Chinese University of Hong Kong, Hong Kong SAR, China
* Correspondence: chongkamlung@cuhk.edu.hk; Tel.: +852-39435859; Fax: +852-27159490

Abstract: Purpose: To elucidate the clinical implications of corneal striae (CS) in thyroid associated orbitopathy (TAO) patients. Methods: In this cross-sectional study, the presence of CS was confirmed after topical fluorescein staining on a slit lamp for consecutive treatment-naive TAO patients. Orbital parameters, including margin reflex distances, lagophthalmos, exophthalmos, intraocular pressure and radiological measurements, were compared between eyes with and without CS. The largest cross-sectional areas of each rectus muscle were measured by segmenting the T1-weighted (T1W) magnetic resonance images (MRI). The logistic regression analyses were used to evaluate the associations between CS and orbital parameters and rectus muscle measurements. Results: Fifty-three consecutive TAO patients (presenting age 46.47 ± 14.73 years, clinical activity score 1.77 ± 1.25) who had unilateral CS were enrolled. In univariate analysis, both the degree of lagophthalmos and the area of the levator palpebrae superioris–superior rectus complex (LPS/SR) on T1W MRI were significantly larger in CS eyes compared to eyes without CS ($p < 0.05$). Multivariate analyses showed that CS in TAO patients were significantly associated with the degree of lagophthalmos (OR = 1.75, 95% CI: 1.18–2.61, $p < 0.05$) and LPS/SR area (OR = 19.27, 95% CI: 1.43–259.32, $p < 0.05$) but not with the other parameters. CS could predict LPS/SR enlargement and larger lagophthalmos in TAO ($p < 0.05$). The largest cross-sectional areas of LPS/SR and inferior rectus were positively correlated with clinical activity scores ($p < 0.05$). Conclusions: The presence of CS in TAO eye is significantly associated with LPS/SR enlargement and worse lagophthalmos. CS might be evaluated further as a potential ocular surface biomarker to identify upper lid and LPS/SR involvement in TAO.

Keywords: thyroid associated orbitopathy; corneal striae; lagophthalmos; extraocular muscle; levator palpebrae superioris–superior rectus complex

Citation: Liao, X.; Aljufairi, F.M.A.A.; Lai, K.K.H.; Chan, K.K.W.; Jia, R.; Chen, W.; Hu, Z.; Wei, Y.; Chu, W.C.W.; Tham, C.C.Y.; et al. Clinical Significance of Corneal Striae in Thyroid Associated Orbitopathy. *J. Clin. Med.* **2023**, *12*, 2284. https://doi.org/10.3390/jcm12062284

Academic Editors: Andrzej Grzybowski and Vito Romano

Received: 3 February 2023
Revised: 6 March 2023
Accepted: 14 March 2023
Published: 15 March 2023

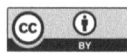

Copyright: © 2023 by the authors. Licensee MDPI, Basel, Switzerland. This article is an open access article distributed under the terms and conditions of the Creative Commons Attribution (CC BY) license (https://creativecommons.org/licenses/by/4.0/).

1. Introduction

Thyroid associated orbitopathy (TAO), also known as thyroid eye disease and Grave's orbitopathy [1], is an autoimmune disorder primarily involving orbital soft tissues. Around 80% of cases are associated with hyperthyroidism [2], and the remaining 20% are associated with either hypothyroidism, Hashimoto's disease or even euthyroidism. TAO is characterized by inflammatory expansion and infiltration of retro-ocular tissues within the orbits, the expansion of adipose tissues within or around the eye muscles and the increase in extraocular muscles and orbital fat chondroitin sulphate and hyaluronan deposition due to excess production of glycosaminoglycan [3]. TAO is often a biphasic disease, which typically begins with an active inflammatory stage that lasts for 12–24 months, followed by a chronic stable fibrotic stage [4,5].

The diagnosis of TAO is essentially based on clinical examinations. The severity of the disease may range from a mild form, which manifests in eyelid and soft tissue involvement, to a very severe form, including sight-threatening globe subluxation, exposure keratopathy [6] and dysthyroid optic neuropathy [7]. These complications often occur due to the delay in diagnosis and treatment. Clinical activity score (CAS) is widely used to grade the inflammatory activity of TAO; a score of 3 or more is considered as active disease. However, patients with low CAS who progressed and developed severe TAO were increasingly reported [8]. Orbital imaging techniques, especially magnetic resonance imaging (MRI), are found useful in quantifying disease activity and severity [9]. However, these modalities are costly, time consuming, and high-quality images are not easily available.

Corneal striae were first reported in an oriental female from a UK group [10] and later by our group in Chinese patients [11]. They are vertical wrinkle-like streaks on the corneal epithelial layer. They are best observed after topical fluorescence staining under cobalt blue light using slit-lamp microscopy (Figure 1), which is simple, non-invasive and widely available in ophthalmology clinics. The clinical implications of corneal striae in TAO remain understudied. Herein, we compare the eyes of the same individual TAO patients who presented with unilateral corneal striae, comparing their orbital and radiological parameters.

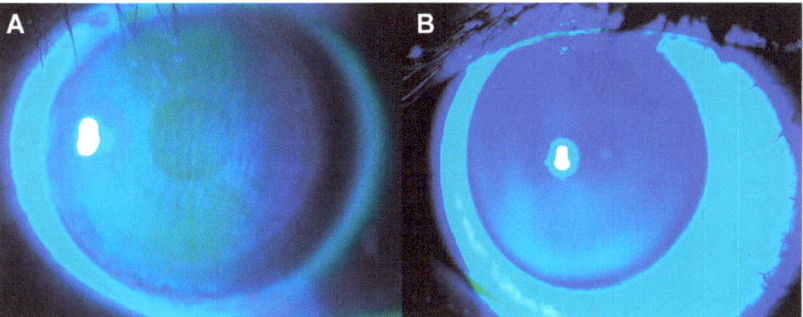

Figure 1. Corneal striae were determined during slit-lamp examination after sodium fluorescence staining. (**A**) Corneal striae in TAO. (**B**) Normal cornea in TAO.

2. Methods

This is a cross-sectional study. Only treatment-naive TAO patients with unilateral corneal striae were analyzed. Patients were consecutively recruited from a TAO cohort of over 1300 Chinese patients in Hong Kong established from 2012 to 2022. The patients were recruited from the Chinese University of Hong Kong Eye Centre, the Eye Centre at the Chinese University of Hong Kong Medical Centre and the Eye Centre at the Prince of Wales Hospital. This study adhered to the tenets of the Declaration of Helsinki and the Ethics approvals (KC/KE-10-0218/ER-3, NTEC Ref. 2010.594) obtained from the Chinese University of Hong Kong. We included patients with clinical diagnoses of TAO presented to a single oculoplastic surgeon [9,12]. We excluded patients with incomplete clinical or radiological data.

2.1. Orbital Examination

The orbital examination included margin reflex distance to the upper eyelid (MRD1), margin reflex distance to the lower eyelid (MRD2), lagophthalmos and clinical activity score (CAS) [13]. The Hertel exophthalmometer was used to measure the degree of exophthalmos [14]. The Goldmann Applanation Tonometer was used to measure the intraocular pressure (IOP) in primary and upgaze [15].

2.2. Magnetic Resonance Imaging

Orbital MRI was arranged for all subjects recruited for this study during their first visit shortly after the initial orbital and slit-lamp examination was performed. MRI was performed using either the 3.0 T Siemens scanner (MAGNETOM Prisma, Siemens, Erlangen, Germany) or the 3.0 T Philips scanner (Achieva TX; Philips Healthcare, Best, The Netherlands). In the 3.0 T Siemens scanner (MAGNETOM Prisma, Siemens, Erlangen, Germany), a 64-channel head/neck coil was used. Coronal T1WI pre-contrast T1-weighted imaging was conducted using the turbo spin echo (TSE) technique at the coronal plane: repetition time (TR)/echo time (TE) = 585/16 ms; acceleration factor for phase encoding (Accel. factor PE) = 3; voxel size = 0.2×0.2 mm; matrix = 384×307; slice thickness = 3.0 mm; slice number = 26; flip angle = $130°$; number of averages = 3. Meanwhile, in the 3.0 T Philips scanner (Achieva TX; Philips Healthcare, Best, the Netherlands), 16-channel Philips neurovascular phased-array coils were used. Coronal T1WI pre-contrast T1-weighted imaging was conducted using the turbo spin echo (TSE) technique at the coronal plane: repetition time (TR)/echo time (TE) = 642/13 ms; TSE factor = 4; slice thickness/gap = 3.0 mm/0.3 mm; slice number = 26; voxel size = 0.3×0.3 mm; matrix = 300×239; flip angle = $90°$; NSA = 1. The type of MRI machine used was largely based on the availability at the MRI center. The patients were instructed to close their eyes and remain motionless during scanning, after stabilizing their heads in a supine position.

T1-weighted (T1W) coronal images were used to measure the cross-sectional area of individual extraocular muscles, which included medial rectus (MR), inferior rectus (IR), lateral rectus (LR) and levator palpebrae superioris–superior rectus complex (LPS/SR). This has been regarded as the best sequence to delineate the orbital muscle anatomy [16]. The coronal section with the largest cross-sectional area for each muscle belly was chosen for measurement. The region of interest (ROI) was manually traced around the surface of each extraocular muscle by a single oculoplastic surgeon who was blinded to the clinical examination findings using a dedicated workstation (Syngo. Via, Siemens, Erlangan, Germany). Each muscle area was measured 3 times, and the mean value was taken (Figure 2).

2.3. Statistical Analyses

The data analyses were performed using the IBM SPSS 23.0 (IBM SPSS Inc., Armonk, NY, USA) and R (The R Project for Statistical Computing, version 4.2.1). Graphs were generated using GraphPad Prism 8.0.1 (GraphPad Software, La Jolla, CA, USA). Continuous variables were described using means ± standard deviations. To compare the difference between two groups, the Chi-square test was used for categorical variables, and the paired t-test was used for continuous variables. The univariate and multivariate logistic regression analyses were used to detect the association between corneal striae and measurement parameters in TAO eyes. The generalized estimating equation was used to correct inter-eye correlation. The ROC curve was used to analyze the effect of IOP, orbital parameters and the area of EOM to differentiate between the eyes with or without corneal striae from each TAO patient. We also applied linear regression analysis to investigate the relationship between the CAS and the largest cross-sectional area of EOM in TAO patients. Results were considered statistically significant if the *p*-value < 0.05.

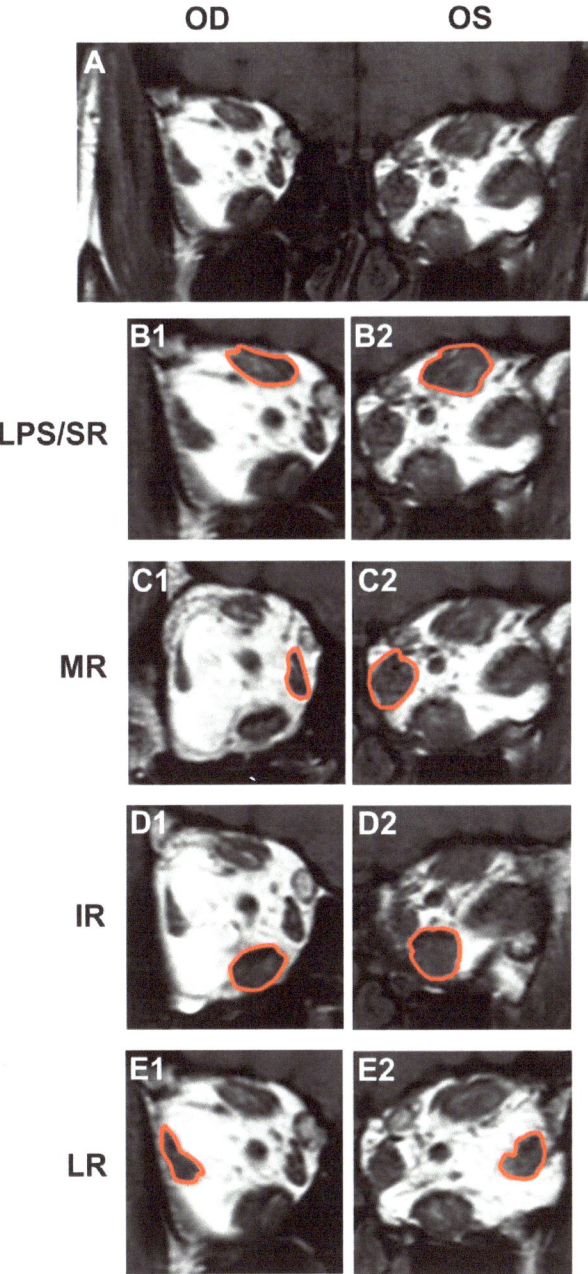

Figure 2. The measurement of the largest cross-sectional area of the extraocular muscle on T1-weighted MR images. (**A**). Representative T1W orbital MR image. (**B1,B2**). Segmentation of the largest LPS/SR image. (**C1,C2**). Segmentation of the largest medial rectus (MR) image. (**D1,D2**). Segmentation of the largest lateral rectus (LR) image. (**E1,E2**). Segmentation of the largest inferior rectus (IR) image. Red line represents segmentation of extraocular muscles. LPS/SR, levator palpebrae superioris–superior rectus complex.

3. Results

Out of our cohort of 1300 patients with TAO, 53 (4.1%) had unilateral corneal striae, and 338 (26.0%) had corneal striae present in at least one eye. In our study, we analyzed a total of 53 TAO patients (106 eyes) with unilateral corneal striae. The mean age at evaluation was 48.83 ± 14.46 years, the age at TAO onset was 46.47 ± 14.73 years, and the clinical activity score presented was 1.77 ± 1.25. Among them, 32.1% (17/53) were smokers, and 92.5% (49/53) had Graves' disease. The demographic characteristics of 53 TAO patients with unilateral corneal striae are summarized in Table 1. It is noted that TAO-related corneal striae are vertically oriented.

Table 1. Demographic characteristics of 53 TAO patients with unilateral corneal striae.

Parameters	Patients with TAO
Number of patients	53
Number of eyes	106
Number of CS eyes (N%)	53 (50%)
Age (years)	48.83 ± 14.46
Female:Male	36:17
Onset age of TAO (years)	46.47 ± 14.73
Clinical activity score	1.77 ± 1.25
Graves' disease (N%)	49 (92.5%)
Smoker (N%)	17 (32.1%)

TAO, thyroid associated orbitopathy; CS, corneal striae.

We found that eyes with corneal striae always had more lagophthalmos (0.83 ± 1.10 mm vs. 0.42 ± 0.69 mm, $p = 0.022$) and larger LPS/SR cross-sectional area (0.52 ± 0.21 cm^2 vs. 0.42 ± 0.21 cm^2, $p = 0.003$) than eyes without corneal striae from the same individual (Table 2).

Table 2. Comparison of measurement results between TAO eyes with and without corneal striae in 53 TAO patients.

	TAO with CS	TAO without CS	p-Value
Number of eyes	53	53	
BCVA (Log MAR)	0.13 ± 0.20	0.08 ± 0.18	0.143
IOP Primary (mmHg)	17.15 ± 3.77	16.94 ± 3.34	0.765
IOP Upgaze (mmHg)	25.53 ± 6.37	24.91 ± 6.56	0.704
Orbital parameters			
MRD1 (mm)	5.60 ± 1.98	5.15 ± 2.06	0.277
MRD2 (mm)	5.15 ± 1.22	5.11 ± 1.12	0.974
Lagophthalmos (mm)	0.83 ± 1.10	0.42 ± 0.69	0.022
Exophthalmos (mm)	18.84 ± 2.43	18.52 ± 2.77	0.484
Extraocular muscles			
LPS/SR (cm^2)	0.52 ± 0.21	0.42 ± 0.21	0.003
Medial rectus (cm^2)	0.36 ± 0.20	0.33 ± 0.13	0.401
Lateral rectus (cm^2)	0.39 ± 0.15	0.41 ± 0.15	0.270
Inferior rectus (cm^2)	0.56 ± 0.25	0.54 ± 0.23	0.845

TAO, thyroid associated orbitopathy; CS, corneal striae; BCVA, best corrected visual acuity; IOP, intraocular pressure; MRD1, margin reflex distance to the upper eyelid; MRD2, margin reflex distance to the lower eyelid; LPS/SR, levator palpebrae superioris–superior rectus complex.

Using univariate logistic regression, the odds ratio of lagophthalmos was found to be 1.69, and the 95% CI was 1.17 to 2.45, with $p = 0.005$. The odds ratio of the cross-sectional area of the LPS/SR was 12.70, and the 95% CI was 1.15 to 140.47, $p = 0.038$ (Table 3).

Table 3. Association of corneal striae and measurement parameters in TAO eyes (N = 106).

	Univariate Model OR (95% CI) p-Value	Multivariate Model * OR (95% CI) p-Value
IOP Primary (mmHg)	1.02 (0.95, 1.09) 0.645	1.02 (0.94, 1.10) 0.646
IOP Upgaze (mmHg)	1.02 (0.98, 1.05) 0.358	1.02 (0.98, 1.05) 0.360
Orbital parameters		
MRD1 (mm)	1.12 (0.98, 1.28) 0.103	1.13 (0.98, 1.32) 0.101
MRD2 (mm)	1.03 (0.85, 1.24) 0.770	1.03 (0.85, 1.25) 0.770
Lagophthalmos (mm)	1.69 (1.17, 2.45) 0.005	1.75 (1.18, 2.61) 0.006
Exophthalmos (mm)	1.05 (0.98, 1.12) 0.172	1.06 (0.98, 1.14) 0.171
Extraocular muscles		
LPS/SR (cm^2)	12.70 (1.15, 140.47) 0.038	19.27 (1.43, 259.32) 0.026
Medial rectus (cm^2)	3.61 (1.00, 12.95) 0.049	5.18 (0.93, 28.94) 0.061
Lateral rectus (cm^2)	0.38 (0.08, 1.87) 0.235	0.31 (0.04, 2.16) 0.238
Inferior rectus (cm^2)	1.43 (0.53, 3.85) 0.474	1.65 (0.42, 6.47) 0.476

TAO, thyroid associated orbitopathy; IOP, intraocular pressure; MRD1, margin reflex distance to the upper eyelid; MRD2, margin reflex distance to the lower eyelid; LPS/SR, levator palpebrae superioris–superior rectus complex. * Multivariate model adjusted for age, sex, Graves' disease, smoker.

After multivariate logistic regression adjusting for age, sex, Graves' disease status and smoking habits, we found that the odds ratio of lagophthalmos was 1.75, and the 95% CI was 1.18 to 2.61, p = 0.006. This was translated into a 75% increase in the risk of developing corneal striae for every 1 mm increase in the degree of lagophthalmos. This also means that among TAO eyes, those with corneal striae had worse lagophthalmos than those without corneal striae. The odds ratio of the cross-sectional area of the LPS/SR was 19.27, and the 95% CI was 1.43 to 259.32, p = 0.026. This indicated that in eyes with TAO, every 1 mm^2 enlargement of the LPS/RS complex was associated with an 18-fold increase in the risk of presenting corneal striae. This also means that in eyes with TAO, those with corneal striae had larger LPS/RS cross-sectional areas than those without corneal striae (Table 3). However, the IOP, MRD, exophthalmos and other EOM enlargements, including the medial rectus, lateral rectus and inferior rectus, did not show significant differences between eyes with and without corneal striae.

The results of the ROC curve analysis showed that the corneal striae could be used as a potential predictive marker for LPS/SR enlargement (area under the ROC curve (AUC) = 0.666, 95% CI = 0.562–0.769, p = 0.001) and lagophthalmos (AUC = 0.598, 95% CI = 0.503–0.692, p = 0.004) in TAO patients (Figure 3 and Table 4).

Table 4. Receiver operating characteristic (ROC) curve analysis of TAO eyes (N = 106).

	AUC	95% CI	p-Value
IOP Primary (mmHg)	0.517	0.406–0.628	0.678
IOP Upgaze (mmHg)	0.479	0.367–0.590	0.390
Orbital parameters			
MRD1 (mm)	0.560	0.452–0.669	0.089
MRD2 (mm)	0.498	0.392–0.604	0.752
Lagophthalmos (mm)	0.598	0.503–0.692	0.004
Exophthalmos (mm)	0.539	0.429–0.650	0.074
Extraocular muscles			
LPS/SR (cm^2)	0.666	0.562–0.769	0.001
Medial rectus (cm^2)	0.547	0.436–0.658	0.179
Lateral rectus (cm^2)	0.562	0.451–0.673	0.305
Inferior rectus (cm^2)	0.511	0.400–0.622	0.227

AUC, area under the ROC curve; IOP, intraocular pressure; MRD1, margin reflex distance to the upper eyelid; MRD2, margin reflex distance to the lower eyelid; LPS/SR, levator palpebrae superioris–superior rectus complex.

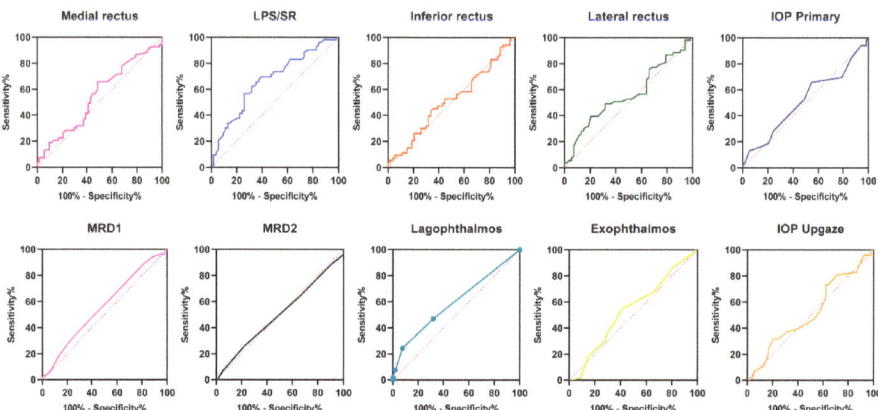

Figure 3. Receiver operating characteristic (ROC) curve analysis showing the area under the curve (AUC) of the diagnostic confidence for different parameters. IOP, intraocular pressure; MRD1, margin reflex distance to the upper eyelid; MRD2, margin reflex distance to the lower eyelid; LPS/SR, levator palpebrae superioris–superior rectus complex.

Linear regression analysis showed that the largest cross-sectional areas of LPS/SR ($r = 0.2566$, $p = 0.0079$) and inferior rectus ($r = 0.2026$, $p = 0.0373$) were positively correlated with the clinical activity score in TAO patients (Figure 4).

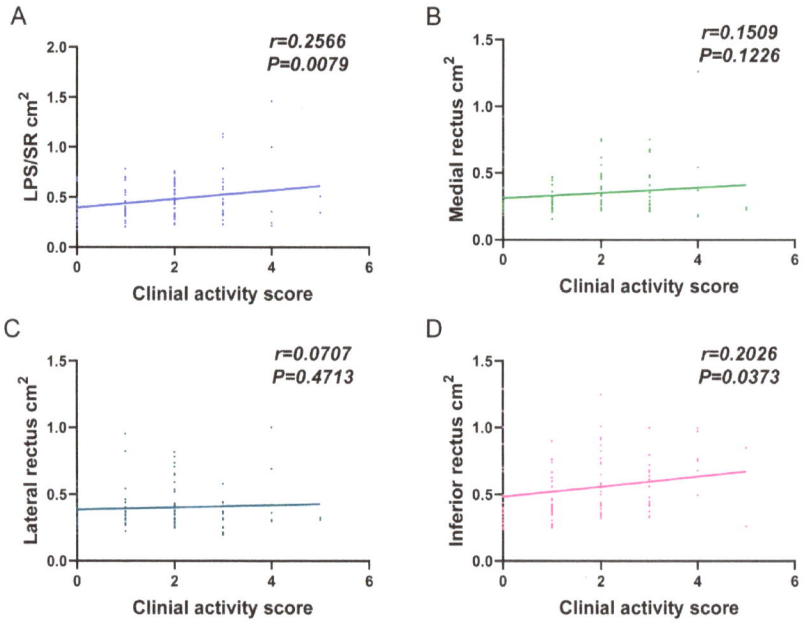

Figure 4. Linear regression analysis of the changes in clinical activity scores and the largest cross-sectional area of extraocular muscles. (**A**) LPS/SR; (**B**) Medial rectus; (**C**) Lateral rectus; (**D**) Inferior rectus) in 53 TAO patients. IOP, intraocular pressure; MRD1, margin reflex distance to the upper eyelid; MRD2, margin reflex distance to the lower eyelid; LPS/SR, levator palpebrae superioris–superior rectus complex.

4. Discussion

Published data on the clinical significance of corneal striae in TAO patients are limited. We noticed reports of corneal striae in two TAO patients [9,10]. Corneal striae were also reported in different ophthalmic diseases, such as primary congenital glaucoma [17], keratoconus [18], Fuchs' endothelial corneal dystrophy [19] and post-LASIK corneal striae [20]. However, corneal striae in our study were only presented vertically, different from the post-LASIK corneal striae with lines resembling fine lattice [20] or Haab's striae with thickened parallel cord-like lines [21]. Our study also showed that the TAO eye with corneal striae was significantly associated with worse lagophthalmos and larger LPS/SR.

Lagophthalmos is the incomplete or defective closure of the eyelids. It is a common manifestation of TAO due to eyelid retraction and/or exophthalmos. On the other hand, it can also present in other eye diseases, such as facial nerve paralysis [22], after trauma or surgery [23]. TAO patients with severe lagophthalmos are prone to increased tear aqueous evaporation, and thus, evaporative dry eye symptoms.

TAO is an autoimmune-driven orbital disease, which results in the infiltration and enlargement of extraocular muscles, orbital fat, eyelid and lacrimal glands. MRI is now increasingly used in TAO to provide an objective evaluation of the inflammatory involvement and/or enlargement of extraocular muscles, lacrimal glands and orbital fat [24]. In this study, we found that for the same TAO patients, the eyes with corneal striae always have larger LPS/SR. An increase in LPS/SR area by 1 mm^2 increases the risk of corneal striae by around 18-fold. Our findings indicate that corneal epithelial changes, readily captured by slit-lamp biomicroscopes, may predict orbital radiological abnormalities, in this case, an enlarged LPS/SR complex. We speculate that the enlargement of the LPS/SR results in undue pressure on the cornea, leading to the development of corneal striae.

Previous studies on corneal striae were associated with abnormal intraocular pressure, especially with low IOP being reported [25,26]. In this study, the IOP (including in primary and upgaze) was not associated with corneal striae. The physiology and biomechanics of corneal striae in TAO need further investigation.

There are many disease markers for TAO, such as serum thyroid-stimulating immunoglobulin (TSI) [27] and orbital images, including MRI [28]. However, in our study, we found that corneal striae, which can be easily observed under a slit lamp, are an indicator of underlying LPS/SR muscle enlargement and upper eyelid involvement. This is useful for identifying patients with a higher likelihood of severe TAO. The presence of corneal striae will help triage patients for earlier assessment by oculoplastic surgeons and/or arrange orbital MR imaging examination for better assessment of disease status.

Our study revealed a positive correlation between the largest cross-sectional area of LPS/SR and the clinical activity score in patients with TAO. We also observed that the enlargement of LPS/SR was related to corneal striae, suggesting a potential positive association between CS and the clinical activity score in TAO patients. Further studies are needed to confirm whether corneal striae alone or in combination may serve as a potential disease marker of TAO severity and activity, as well as the biomechanical basis of corneal striae. Additionally, further research is needed to determine whether CS will disappear after treatment with decompression surgery, eyelid surgery or lubricating eye drops. There are logistic merits to evaluating corneal striae under a slit lamp; namely, it is a simple, non-invasive and readily available technique in eye clinics.

In conclusion, we comprehensively studied a "new" clinical feature in TAO patients, the corneal striae. Our results showed that corneal striae are vertical and significantly associated with worse lagophthalmos and larger LPS/SR cross-sectional area. Corneal striae might be evaluated as a non-invasive biomarker to determine TAO severity and activity.

Author Contributions: Methodology, F.M.A.A.A., K.K.H.L., K.K.W.C. and W.C.W.C.; Software, Z.H.; Investigation, W.C.; Resources, C.C.Y.T. and C.P.P.; Data curation, R.J. and Y.W.; Writing—original draft, X.L.; Project administration, K.K.L.C. All authors have read and agreed to the published version of the manuscript.

Funding: This study was supported in part by S.K. Yee Medical Foundation, Hong Kong (Project no. 2191216) and the General Research Fund, Research Grants Council, Hong Kong (Grant no. 14103221).

Institutional Review Board Statement: This study was approved by the Ethics Committee of the Chinese University of Hong Kong and performed in accordance with the tenets of the Declaration of Helsinki (KC/KE-10-0218/ER-3, NTEC Ref. 2010.594).

Informed Consent Statement: Informed consent was obtained from all subjects involved in the study.

Data Availability Statement: Not applicable.

Conflicts of Interest: The authors declare no conflict of interest.

References

1. Bahn, R.S. Graves' Ophthalmopathy. *N. Engl. J. Med.* **2010**, *362*, 726–738. [CrossRef] [PubMed]
2. Cockerham, K.P.; Chan, S.S. Thyroid Eye Disease. *Neurol. Clin.* **2010**, *28*, 729–755. [CrossRef] [PubMed]
3. Lee, A.C.H.; Kahaly, G.J. Pathophysiology of thyroid-associated orbitopathy. *Best Pract. Res. Clin. Endocrinol. Metab.* **2022**, 101620. [CrossRef] [PubMed]
4. Wang, Y.; Smith, T.J. Current Concepts in the Molecular Pathogenesis of Thyroid-Associated Ophthalmopathy. *Investig. Ophthalmol. Vis. Sci.* **2014**, *55*, 1735–1748. [CrossRef] [PubMed]
5. Fang, S.; Huang, Y.; Wang, S.; Zhang, Y.; Luo, X.; Liu, L.; Zhong, S.; Liu, X.; Li, D.; Liang, R.; et al. IL-17A Exacerbates Fibrosis by Promoting the Proinflammatory and Profibrotic Function of Orbital Fibroblasts in TAO. *J. Clin. Endocrinol. Metab.* **2016**, *101*, 2955–2965. [CrossRef] [PubMed]
6. Alsuhaibani, A.H.; Nerad, J.A. Thyroid-Associated Orbitopathy. *Semin. Plast. Surg.* **2007**, *21*, 065–073. [CrossRef]
7. Ji, X.; Xiao, W.; Ye, H.; Chen, R.; Wu, J.; Mao, Y.; Yang, H. Ultrasonographic measurement of the optic nerve sheath diameter in dysthyroid optic neuropathy. *Eye* **2021**, *35*, 568–574. [CrossRef]
8. Iñiguez-Ariza, N.M.; Sharma, A.; Garrity, J.A.; Stan, M.N. The "Quiet TED"—A Special Subgroup of Thyroid Eye Disease. *Ophthalmic Plast. Reconstr. Surg.* **2021**, *37*, 551–555. [CrossRef]
9. Bartalena, L.; Kahaly, G.J.; Baldeschi, L.; Dayan, C.M.; Eckstein, A.; Marcocci, C.; Marinò, M.; Vaidya, B.; Wiersinga, W.M.; Ayvaz, G.; et al. The 2021 European Group on Graves' orbitopathy (EUGOGO) clinical practice guidelines for the medical management of Graves' orbitopathy. *Eur. J. Endocrinol.* **2021**, *185*, G43–G67. [CrossRef]
10. Kashani, S.; Papadopoulos, R.; Olver, J. Corneal striae in thyroid eye disease. *Eye* **2007**, *21*, 869–870. [CrossRef]
11. Lam, C.C.; Chong, K.K. Spontaneous intercalated corneal epithelial folds in thyroid eye disease: A case report. *Hong Kong J. Ophthalmol.* **2020**, *24*, 60–62. [CrossRef]
12. Bartley, G.B.; Gorman, C.A. Diagnostic Criteria for Graves' Ophthalmopathy. *Am. J. Ophthalmol.* **1995**, *119*, 792–795. [CrossRef] [PubMed]
13. Lee, D.C.; Young, S.M.; Kim, Y.-D.; Woo, K.I. Course of upper eyelid retraction in thyroid eye disease. *Br. J. Ophthalmol.* **2020**, *104*, 254–259. [CrossRef]
14. Kozaki, A.; Inoue, R.; Komoto, N.; Maeda, T.; Inoue, Y.; Inoue, T.; Ayaki, M. Proptosis in Dysthyroid Ophthalmopathy: A Case Series of 10,931 Japanese Cases. *Optom. Vis. Sci.* **2010**, *87*, 200–204. [CrossRef]
15. Feizi, S.; Faramarzi, A.; Kheiri, B. Goldmann applanation tonometer versus ocular response analyzer for measuring intraocular pressure after congenital cataract surgery. *Eur. J. Ophthalmol.* **2018**, *28*, 582–589. [CrossRef]
16. Ma, R.; Geng, Y.; Gan, L.; Peng, Z.; Cheng, J.; Guo, J.; Qian, J. Quantitative T1 mapping MRI for the assessment of extraocular muscle fibrosis in thyroid-associated ophthalmopathy. *Endocrine* **2022**, *75*, 456–464. [CrossRef]
17. Tamçelik, N.; Oto, B.B.; Mergen, B.; Kiliçarslan, O.; Gönen, B.; Arici, C. Corneal Endothelial Changes in Patients With Primary Congenital Glaucoma. *J. Glaucoma* **2022**, *31*, 123–128. [CrossRef]
18. Rakhshandadi, T.; Sedaghat, M.-R.; Askarizadeh, F.; Momeni-Moghaddam, H.; Khabazkhoob, M.; Yekta, A.; Narooie-Noori, F. Refractive characteristics of keratoconus eyes with corneal Vogt's striae: A contralateral eye study. *J. Optom.* **2021**, *14*, 183–188. [CrossRef]
19. Thuret, G.; Ain, A.; Koizumi, N.; Okumura, N.; Gain, P.; He, Z. Radial Endothelial Striae over 360 Degrees in Fuchs Corneal Endothelial Dystrophy: New Pathophysiological Findings. *Cornea* **2021**, *40*, 1604–1606. [CrossRef] [PubMed]
20. Donnenfeld, E.D.; Perry, H.D.; Doshi, S.J.; Biser, S.A.; Solomon, R. Hyperthermic treatment of post-LASIK corneal striae. *J. Cataract. Refract. Surg.* **2004**, *30*, 620–625. [CrossRef]
21. Mandal, A.K.; Raghavachary, C.; Peguda, H.K. Haab's Striae. *Ophthalmology* **2017**, *124*, 11. [CrossRef] [PubMed]
22. Tao, J.P.; Vemuri, S.; Patel, A.D.; Compton, C.; Nunery, W.R. Lateral Tarsoconjunctival Onlay Flap Lower Eyelid Suspension in Facial Nerve Paresis. *Ophthalmic Plast. Reconstr. Surg.* **2014**, *30*, 342–345. [CrossRef] [PubMed]
23. Pereira, M.V.C.; Glória, A.L.F. Lagophthalmos. *Semin. Ophthalmol.* **2010**, *25*, 72–78. [CrossRef] [PubMed]
24. Yu, W.; Zheng, L.; Shuo, Z.; Xingtong, L.; Mengda, J.; Lin, Z.; Ziyang, S.; Huifang, Z. Evaluation of extraocular muscles in patients with thyroid associated ophthalmopathy using apparent diffusion coefficient measured by magnetic resonance imaging before and after radiation therapy. *Acta Radiol.* **2021**, *63*, 1180–1186. [CrossRef] [PubMed]

25. Abualhasan, H.; Mimouni, M.; Safuri, S.; Blumenthal, E.Z. Anterior Corneal Folds Correlate With Low Intraocular Pressure and May Serve as a Marker for Ocular Hypotony. *J. Glaucoma* **2019**, *28*, 178–180. [CrossRef] [PubMed]
26. Birnbaum, F.A.; Mirzania, D.; Swaminathan, S.S.; Davis, A.R.; Perez, V.L.; Herndon, L.W. Risk Factors for Corneal Striae in Eyes After Glaucoma Surgery. *J. Glaucoma* **2022**, *31*, 116–122. [CrossRef]
27. Thia, B.; McGuinness, M.B.; Ebeling, P.R.; Khong, J.J. Diagnostic accuracy of Immulite® TSI immunoassay for thyroid-associated orbitopathy in patients with recently diagnosed Graves' hyperthyroidism. *Int. Ophthalmol.* **2022**, *42*, 863–870. [CrossRef]
28. Das, T.; Roos, J.C.P.; Patterson, A.J.; Graves, M.J.; Murthy, R. T2-relaxation mapping and fat fraction assessment to objectively quantify clinical activity in thyroid eye disease: An initial feasibility study. *Eye* **2019**, *33*, 235–243. [CrossRef]

Disclaimer/Publisher's Note: The statements, opinions and data contained in all publications are solely those of the individual author(s) and contributor(s) and not of MDPI and/or the editor(s). MDPI and/or the editor(s) disclaim responsibility for any injury to people or property resulting from any ideas, methods, instructions or products referred to in the content.

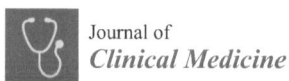 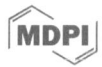

Article

Incidence of Orbital Side Effects in Zygomaticomaxillary Complex and Isolated Orbital Walls Fractures: A Retrospective Study in South Italy and a Brief Review of the Literature

Umberto Committeri [1,*], Antonio Arena [1], Emanuele Carraturo [1], Martina Austoni [1], Cristiana Germano [1], Giovanni Salzano [2], Giacomo De Riu [3], Francesco Giovacchini [4], Fabio Maglitto [1], Vincenzo Abbate [1], Paola Bonavolontà [1], Luigi Califano [1] and Pasquale Piombino [1]

[1] Maxillofacial Surgery Unit, Department of Neurosciences, Reproductive and Odontostomatological Sciences, University of Naples "Federico II", 80131 Naples, Italy
[2] Otolaryngology and Maxillo-Facial Surgery Unit, Istituto Nazionale Tumori—IRCCS Fondazione G. Pascale, 80131 Naples, Italy
[3] Maxillofacial Surgery Operative Unit, University Hospital of Sassari, 07100 Sassari, Italy
[4] Maxillofacial Surgery Unit, Santa Maria Della Misericordia Hospital, San Sisto, 06121 Perugia, Italy
* Correspondence: umbertocommitteri@gmail.com; Tel.: +39-340-307-8637

Citation: Committeri, U.; Arena, A.; Carraturo, E.; Austoni, M.; Germano, C.; Salzano, G.; De Riu, G.; Giovacchini, F.; Maglitto, F.; Abbate, V.; et al. Incidence of Orbital Side Effects in Zygomaticomaxillary Complex and Isolated Orbital Walls Fractures: A Retrospective Study in South Italy and a Brief Review of the Literature. J. Clin. Med. 2023, 12, 845. https://doi.org/10.3390/jcm12030845

Academic Editor: Atsushi Mizota

Received: 5 December 2022
Revised: 4 January 2023
Accepted: 16 January 2023
Published: 20 January 2023

Correction Statement: This article has been republished with a minor change. The change does not affect the scientific content of the article and further details are available within the backmatter of the website version of this article.

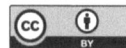

Copyright: © 2023 by the authors. Licensee MDPI, Basel, Switzerland. This article is an open access article distributed under the terms and conditions of the Creative Commons Attribution (CC BY) license (https://creativecommons.org/licenses/by/4.0/).

Abstract: Zygomaticomaxillary complex and isolated orbital walls fractures are one of the most common fractures of the midface, often presenting orbital symptoms and complications. Our study was born with the aim of understanding the trend in the incidence of orbital presurgical symptoms, specifically diplopia, enophthalmos and exophthalmos, in the Campania Region in southern Italy. We conducted a retrospective, monocentric observational study at the Maxillofacial Surgery Unit of the Federico II University Hospital of Naples, enrolling 402 patients who reported a fracture of the zygomaticomaxillary complex and orbital floor region from 1 January 2012 to 1 January 2022. Patients were evaluated by age, gender, etiology, type of fracture, preoperative orbital side effects and symptoms. Pre-surgical side effects were studied, and 16% of patients ($n = 66$) developed diplopia. Diplopia was most common in patients previously operated on for orbital wall fractures (100%), and least common in patients who reported trauma after interpersonal violence (15%) and road traffic accidents (11%). Exophthalmos appeared only in 1% (six cases); whereas it did not appear in 99% (396 cases). Enophthalmos was present in 4% (sixteen cases), most commonly in interpersonal violence cases (two cases). The frequency of orbital complications in patients with zygomaticomaxillary complex and isolated orbital walls fractures suggests how diplopia remains the most common pre-surgical orbital side effect.

Keywords: diplopia; zygomaticomaxillary complex fractures; isolated orbital walls fractures; orbit; enophtalmos; exophtalmos

1. Introduction

In the field of cranio-maxillofacial traumatology, zygomaticomaxillary complex and isolated orbital walls fractures are one of the most common fractures of the midface, and account for around 27% of all facial fractures, being second only to nasal fractures [1]. Injury patterns may be isolated to the orbit or form part of a much larger zygomatic-maxillary complex (ZMC) or pan-facial fracture patterns. These fractures are usually classified as pure and impure. Impure orbital fractures are those that involve the orbital rim(s) with the internal orbit walls. Most orbital pure fractures occur along the floor and/or medial walls of the orbit, where the walls are the thinnest [2,3]. Orbital wall fractures are also classified as isolated fractures, involving a single orbital wall, or as combined fractures, when more than one orbital wall is affected [4]. Following the anatomical region of the fracture rim, orbital fractures can be divided into orbital floor, orbital roof, median and lateral wall fractures; the floor is the most frequently injured because it contains the largest open space and lacks support. The frequency of orbital fractures has become more common owing to the increasing amount of traffic accidents, industrial accidents, sport-related injuries and physical assaults, and, rarely, gunshots [5–7]. Management and treatment of orbital fractures poses a challenge to every surgeon and physician in general. This is because of their complex anatomy and their innate relationship to relevant structures, such as the globe, optic nerve and ophthalmic artery, among others, and their direct influence on the most precious of senses: vision. For this reason, they represent the few real urgencies in the realm of Cranio-Maxillofacial trauma [8]. Orbital symptoms are a relatively common complication of orbital fractures. In the medical literature, they occur in about 20% of patients, most frequently in the subgroup of orbital blow fractures. Diagnosis is essential to permit early treatment, as various symptoms, such as diplopia and enophthalmos, may persist even after surgical treatment, especially if the diagnosis is delayed [9,10]. This epidemiological study was born with the aim of understanding the trend in the incidence of orbital presurgical symptoms, specifically diplopia, enophthalmos and exophthalmos, in the Campania Region in southern Italy to help the development of a trauma patient protocol based on the clinical presentation and specific demands.

2. Materials and Methods

The study was conducted at the Maxillofacial Surgery Unit of the Federico II University Hospital, Regional Referral Center for Cranio-Maxillo-Facial Traumas (Article 1 paragraph 203 L.F. Campania Region 2011, Italy). It was a retrospective, monocentric observational study. The sample size consisted of 402 patients who reported a fracture of the zygomaticomaxillary complex and orbital floor. All clinical investigations and procedures were conducted according to the principles expressed in the Declaration of Helsinki. Ethical approval to access and use the data was obtained from the Federico II/Cardarelli Research Ethic Committee (81/2022). Patients were evaluated by age, gender, etiology, type of fracture, preoperative orbital side effects and symptoms. Blind/visually impaired patients, patients suffering from osteoporosis/osteomalacia or psychiatric disorders were excluded. Patients admitted in this study did not suffer from any globe injuries, the management of which would take priority over any maxillofacial procedures. All data were extrapolated from medical records from 1 January 2012 to 1 January 2022 and analyzed in a period of time which goes from 15 June 2021 to 15 June 2022. Definitive diagnosis was obtained by performing computed tomography (CT) (Figure 1).

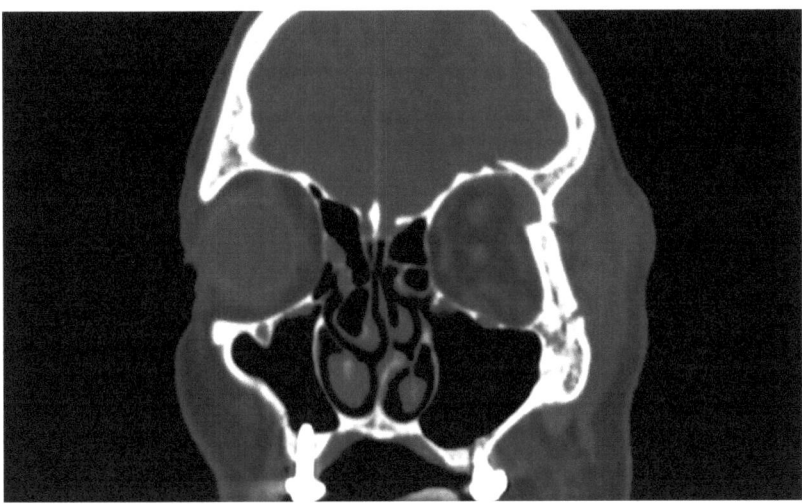

Figure 1. CT scan of a case of diplopia in a patient with a lateral orbit wall fracture.

Preoperative side effects (diplopia, enophtalmos, exophthalmos) were evaluated through accurate ophthalmic clinical examinations by the same operator and using the same instrument (Hertel Exophthalmometer, © 2022 Lombart Instrument, Inc. All Rights Reserved. 800-LOMBART, 5358 Robin Hood Road, Norfolk, Virginia 23513). In the same way, all patients took the Hess-Lancaster screen or Hess-Lancaster red-green test to better diagnose any defect in ocular motility. The considered variables were summarized considering frequency and percentage for each category.

3. Results

The most affected patients were men, representing 77% of the total number of cases (out of a sample of 308 men and 94 women). The most represented age group was between 13–25 years with 22% (90 cases), followed by the 25–37 age group with 19% (76 cases), the 37–49 age group (76 cases) with 19%, the 49–61 age group with 16% (64 cases), the 61–73 age group with 12% (48 cases), the 73–85 age group with 8% (34 cases), and, finally, the 85–97 age group with 3% (14 cases). The mean age reported was 46 years.

From the data obtained, we analyzed the mechanism of the trauma that caused the fracture. In our series, the most frequent causes were accidental falls in 37% (148 cases), road accidents in 36% (144 cases) and interpersonal violence in 16% (66 cases). Among the minor causes, on the other hand, syncopal episodes were found in 4% (sixteen cases), sports accidents in 2% (ten cases), previous fracture outcomes in 3% of cases (fourteen cases), and, finally, 1% were workplace accidents (four cases). From the analyzed data, we noticed that mostly women reported accidental falls, in 60% of cases, and reported road accidents in 30%. Men mostly reported having road accidents (37%), then accidental falls (30%), followed by interpersonal violence (21%).

The fractures were stratified according to the presence or absence of the involvement of the orbital frame, as impure in 64% (258 cases) and in pure in 36% (144 cases), with a frequency ratio of 1.8:1.

These fractures were then further classified according to the area of impact (Figure 2):

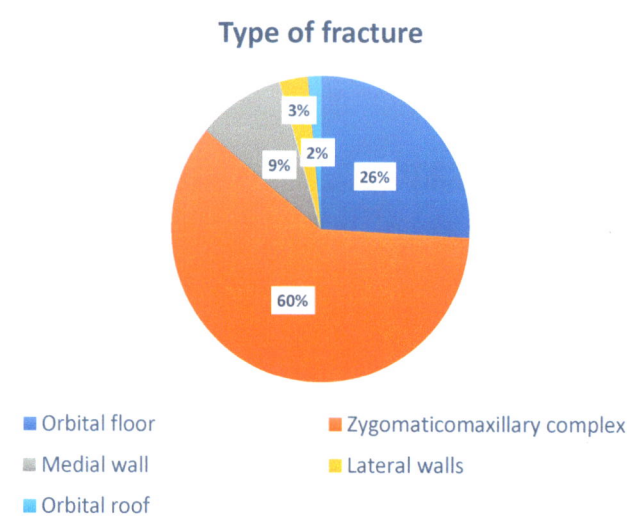

Figure 2. Type of fracture.

- Zygomatic orbital fractures, the most frequent, in 60% (242 cases)
- Fractures of the orbital floor in 26% (104 cases)
- Fractures of the medial wall in 9% (38 cases)

- Fractures of the lateral wall in 3% (12 cases)
- Fractures of the orbital roof in 1% (6 cases)

Among the orbital side effects, we found the following (Figure 3):

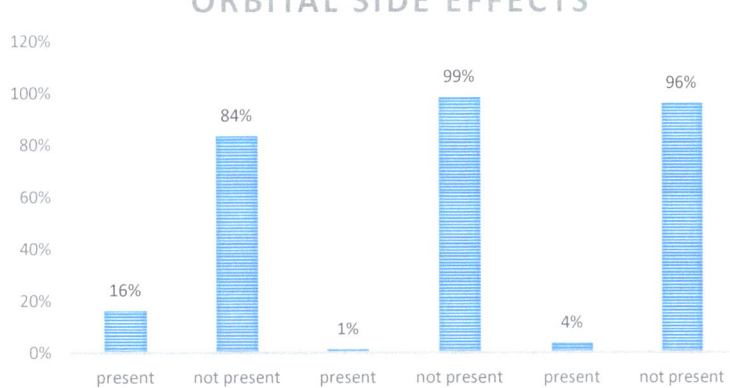

Figure 3. Orbital side effects.

Diplopia: 84% of patients did not report double vision (336 cases), 16% reported diplopia (66 cases).

Exophthalmos appeared only in 1% (6 cases), while it did not appear in 99% (396 cases).

Enophthalmos was present in 4% (16 cases), while it was not present in 96% (386 cases).

Correlating the type of fracture with the orbital side effects (Table 1), we found, that among orbital floor fractures, 42% of patients reported diplopia ($n = 44$); in 17% of lateral wall fractures diplopia ($n = 2$) was reported, in 16% of medial wall fractures diplopia ($n = 6$) was reported, and in 6% of zygomaticomaxillary fractures diplopia ($n = 14$) was reported.

Table 1. Correlation between fractures and orbital side effects.

Type of Fracture	Number of Fractures	Diplopia%
Orbital floor	104	42%
Zygomaticomaxillary complex	242	6%
Medial wall	38	16%
Lateral walls	12	17%
Orbital roof	6	0%
Type of Fracture	**Number of Fractures**	**Exhophtalmos%**
Orbital floor	104	2%
Zygomaticomaxillary complex	242	2%
Medial wall	38	0%
Lateral walls	12	0%
Orbital roof	6	0%
Type of Fracture	**Number of Fractures**	**Enophtalmos%**
Orbital floor	104	10%
Zygomaticomaxillary complex	242	1%
Medial wall	38	11%
Lateral walls	12	0%
Orbital roof	6	0%

Considering exophthalmos, it was found in 2% of orbital floor fractures ($n = 2$) and in 2% of zygomaticomaxillary fractures ($n = 4$).

Enophthalmos was reported in 10% of orbital floor fractures ($n = 10$), and in 11% of medial orbital wall fractures ($n = 4$).

Correlating the cause of the trauma and the orbital complications (Figure 4), it was found that, in the studied cohort, 100% of diplopia cases were present in patients who had previously undergone surgery for orbital wall fractures ($n = 14$), 40% while practicing sports ($n = 4$), 15% occurred in interpersonal violence cases ($n = 10$), 14% in accidental fall cases ($n = 20$), 13% in syncopal episode cases ($n = 10$) and 11% in road traffic accident ($n = 16$), while none occurred in a workplace setting.

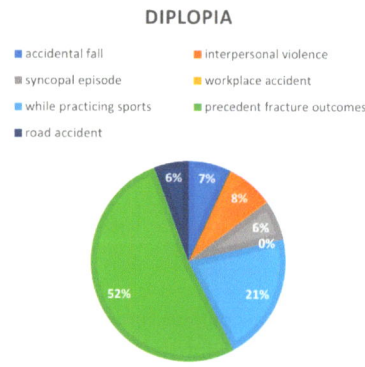

Figure 4. Diplopia correlated to cause of the fractures.

Exophthalmos in the considered cohort (Figure 5) were present in 8% of syncopal episodes cases ($n = 2$), 3% in interpersonal violence cases ($n = 2$) and in 1.3% of road traffic accidents ($n = 2$).

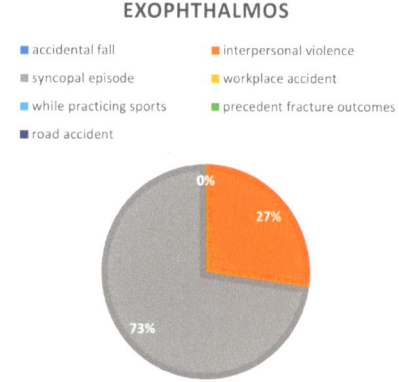

Figure 5. Exophthalmos correlated to cause of the fractures.

Enophthalmos (Figure 6) were present in 42% of patients who had previously undergone surgery for orbital wall fractures ($n = 6$), 12% in interpersonal violence cases ($n = 8$) and in 1.3% of accidental falls ($n = 2$).

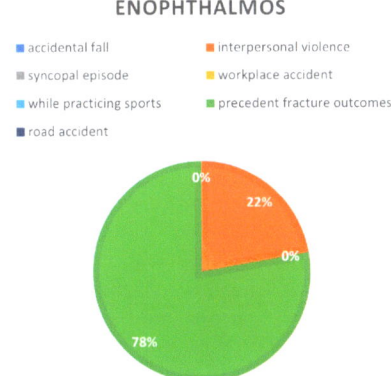

Figure 6. Enophthalmos correlated to cause of the fractures.

4. Discussion

Fractures of the orbitozygomaticomaxillary complex are among the most common fractures of the midface and account for approximately 27% of all facial fractures. Impure orbital fractures are more common than pure orbital fractures [1,2,11].

Isolated orbital wall fractures account for 4% to 16% [3,12].

Early recognition of ocular injuries is fundamental in mid-facial fracture cases. The management of globe injuries often takes precedence over the treatment of mid-facial and orbital fractures. Every surgeon who addresses orbital trauma must consider how to handle an emergency surgery, whereas the fracture pattern leads to optical nerve damage and then vision loss [13].

Diagnosis is essential to permit early treatment, as various symptoms, such as diplopia and enophthalmos, may persist even after surgical treatment, especially if the diagnosis is delayed [4,14]. It is always necessary to ascertain the mechanism that caused the lesion and to reconstruct the patient's medical history before performing a clinical examination of the orbit and globe. The initial ophthalmological assessment should include periorbital examination, visual acuity, ocular motility, pupillary responses, visual fields and a fundoscopic examination [14].

Exophthalmometry is used to measure the position of the globe, while graphic radiographic visualization with coronal CT makes it possible to detail soft tissue not visible with conventional X-rays; Coronal CT scans of 1.5 to 3 mm visualize antral soft tissue densities, such as prolapsed orbital fat, extraocular muscle and hematoma [15].

Diplopia is one of the most common post-traumatic symptoms of orbital fractures [14]. Post-traumatic monocular diplopia can be caused by extrusion of the extraocular muscles or orbital soft tissue, injury to the extraocular muscles, edema of the infraorbital adipose tissue or vertical deviation of the eyeball [16]. Any change in orbital volume directly impacts the position of the globe and its anteroposterior projection and super-inferior position. Enophthalmos can be defined as the displacement of the eyeball in a posterior direction and is attributed to an increase in the intra-orbital volume, while the term exophthalmos refers to a forward displacement of the eyeball [17].

The aim of the study conducted was to show the epidemiological distribution of pre-operative orbital symptoms (diplopia, enophthalmos and exophthalmos) presented by patients who suffered from zygomaticomaxillary complex or isolated orbital wall fractures enrolled in the Oral and Maxillofacial Operative Unit of AOU "Federico II".

The results found in this study agree with the literature, as zygomaticomaxillary complex and isolated orbital walls fractures are the most frequent midface maxillofacial trauma [8,18]. Indeed, 60% (n = 242) of the 402 patients involved in this study had a zygomaticomaxillary complex fracture.

The male/female ratio was 3,4:1, with male involvement representing 77% of total cases, with a mean age reported at 46 years. The fractures were stratified according to the presence or absence of the engagement of the orbital frame, as impure in 64% (258 cases) and as pure in 36% (144 cases), with a frequency ratio of 1.8:1; therefore, the incidence is comparable to other clinical studies [11].

In our series, the most common cause was represented by accidental falls, with 148 cases (37% of the total), 92 of which were men and 56 were women. From the analyzed data, we noticed that mostly women reported accidental falls, with 60% among female cases, and then road accidents with 30%. Men mostly reported having road accidents (37%), accidental falls (30%), followed by interpersonal violence (21%). Among the minor causes, on the other hand, syncopal episodes were found in 4% of cases, sports accidents in 2%, previous fracture outcomes in 3% of cases and, finally, 1% were workplace accidents. This result may be related to a greater tendency in the Campania region to use private means of transport compared to public transport. This trend has been found in similar studies conducted in other Western countries, where it is common for a family to own at least one motor vehicle [19].

In our series, we noted sixty-six patients suffering from pre-operative diplopia (16% of the sample), six patients affected with exophthalmos (1% of the sample) and sixteen patients suffering from enophthalmos (4% of the sample). These findings are not completely supported by the literature, as Bartoli et al. reported diplopia to be a main preoperative complication in 20.2% of patients, followed by enophthalmos (2.3%) and exophthalmos (1.7%), whereas Shin et al. stated diplopia was present in 42.3% of patients [18].

In our sample, 42% of patients suffering from preoperative diplopia reported an orbital floor fracture, while 6% reported diplopia suffering from zygomaticomaxillary complex fractures; 16% had medial wall fractures and 17% had lateral wall fractures. No patients with orbital roof fractures reported diplopia. These outcomes agree with most of the international literature that reported orbital floor fractures as typically coinciding with preoperative diplopia. Ramphul et al. (2017), in their review of 126 patients with orbital floor fractures, underlined that 66.6% of the total sample suffered from preoperative diplopia [20]. A study by Burm et al. included 82 cases and reported that diplopia was associated with 25% of medial wall fractures, 80% of orbital floor fractures and 80.9% of combined medial and floor fractures [21]. Higashino et al. reported 106 cases and showed that 21.4% of medial wall fractures and 23.5% of orbital floor fractures were associated with diplopia [22]. Eun et al. reported on 387 cases in which diplopia was found on physical examination prior to surgery in 22% of medial wall fractures, 78% of floor fractures and 82% of combined medial and floor fractures [23]. Tahiri et al. reported that patients with preoperative diplopia had a 9.91 times greater postoperative risk of persistent diplopia [24].

Our results indicated that 2% of patients with orbital floor fractures showed exophthalmos and another 10% of patients with orbital floor fracture displayed enophthalmos; 2% of patients with zygomatic-maxillary complex fracture exhibited exophthalmos, 1% of presented enophthalmos and no patients with orbital roof, midwall or lateral wall fractures presented exophthalmos. An interesting observation was that enophthalmos, while it was absent in patients with orbital roof and lateral wall fractures (as exophthalmos), was found in 11% of patients with midwall fractures.

The symptoms of medial orbital wall fractures are usually less severe than those of inferior wall fractures because less muscle incarceration takes place, and the bony structure is multiply overlapped [25]. Since medial orbital wall fractures are often asymptomatic, they have received less attention in the literature [26]. However, they may cause complications such as diplopia, enophthalmos and the entrapment of extraocular muscles [27]. In particular, enophthalmos may not immediately appear after the trauma because soft tissue swelling can last weeks or months [28,29]. The international literature shows how medial wall fracture is directly correlated with enophthalmos [30].

Correlating the cause of the fracture with the pre-surgical orbital symptoms, in this study, it was found that 100% of patients who previously underwent surgery for orbital wall fractures presented diplopia, while 38% reported enophthalmos, 40% of patients who experienced trauma while practicing sports reported diplopia and none reported exophthalmos or enophthalmos.

Additionally, 15% of patients who reported an interpersonal violence accident were described as having diplopia, 33% had exophthalmos and 50% had enophthalmos.

In accidental fall cases, 14% of patients described having diplopia, 13% had enophthalmos and none described suffering from exophthalmos.

Cases correlated with syncopal falls reported diplopia in 13% of cases, and 33% reported exophthalmos.

Over a period of 1 year, 402 patients who sustained a fracture in the zygomaticomaxillary complex and isolated orbital walls fractures received a full ophthalmological examination within 1 week of injury.

5. Conclusions

A total of 60% ($n = 242$) of patients enrolled in this study had a zygomaticomaxillary complex fracture and 26% (104 cases) had an orbital floor fracture.

Pre-surgical side effects were studied, and 16% of patients ($n = 66$) developed diplopia. Diplopia was most common in patients who had previously undergone surgery for orbital wall fractures (100%), and was least common in those who had experienced interpersonal violence (15%) and road traffic accidents (11%). Exophthalmos only appeared in 1%, whereas it did not appear in 99% of patients. Enophthalmos was present in 4% of patients, and was more common in interpersonal violence cases.

The frequency of orbital complications in patients with zygomaticomaxillary complex and isolated orbital walls fractures complex has never been assessed before in the literature, and our findings suggest that, in patients under evaluation for orbital trauma, the observation of diplopia remains the most common orbital side effect before surgery.

Author Contributions: Conceptualization, P.P. and F.M.; methodology, U.C. and G.S.; software, E.C. and F.G.; validation, P.P., C.G. and F.M.; formal analysis, M.A.; investigation, E.C.; resources, A.A.; data curation, E.C.; writing—original draft preparation, E.C., V.A. and P.B.; writing—review and editing, P.B., A.A. and U.C.; visualization, G.D.R.; supervision, L.C.; project administration, L.C.; funding acquisition, none. All authors have read and agreed to the published version of the manuscript.

Funding: This research received no external funding.

Institutional Review Board Statement: The study was conducted in accordance with the Declaration of Helsinki, and approved by the Institutional Review Board (or Ethics Committee) of Federico II/Cardarelli Research Ethic Committee (81/2022, 14 April 2022).

Informed Consent Statement: Written informed consent has been obtained from the patient(s) to publish this paper.

Data Availability Statement: The data are available upon request from the corresponding author.

Conflicts of Interest: The authors declare no conflict of interest.

References

1. Jho Johnson, N.R.; Singh, N.R.; Oztel, M.; Vangaveti, V.N.; Rahmel, B.B.; Ramalingam, L. Ophthalmological injuries associated with fractures of the orbitozygomaticomaxillary complex. *Br. J. Oral Maxillofac. Surg.* **2018**, *56*, 221–226. [CrossRef] [PubMed]
2. Converse, J.M.; Smith, B. Blowout fracture of the floor of the orbit. *Trans. Am. Acad. Ophthalmol. Otolaryngol.* **1960**, *64*, 676–688. [PubMed]
3. Cornelius, C.P.; Mayer, P.; Ehrenfeld, M.; Metzger, M.C. The orbits—Anatomical features in view of innovative surgical methods. *Facial Plast. Surg.* **2014**, *30*, 487–508. [CrossRef] [PubMed]
4. Burnstine, M.A. Clinical recommendations for repair of isolated orbital floor fractures: An evidence-based analysis. *Ophthalmology* **2002**, *109*, 1207–1210. [CrossRef] [PubMed]

5. Shin, J.W.; Lim, J.S.; Yoo, G.; Byeon, J.H. An analysis of pure blowout fractures and associated ocular symptoms. *J. Craniofac. Surg.* **2013**, *24*, 703–707. [CrossRef] [PubMed]
6. Tong, L.; Bauer, R.J.; Buchman, S.R. A current 10-year retrospective survey of 199 surgically treated orbital floor fractures in a nonurban tertiary care center. *Plast. Reconstr. Surg.* **2001**, *108*, 612–621. [CrossRef]
7. Turvey, T.A.; Golden, B.A. Orbital anatomy for the surgeon. *Oral. Maxillofac. Surg. Clin. N. Am.* **2012**, *24*, 525–536. [CrossRef]
8. Parameswaran, A.; Marimuthu, M.; Panwar, S.; Hammer, B. Orbital Fractures. In *Oral and Maxillofacial Surgery for the Clinician*; Bonanthaya, K., Panneerselvam, E., Manuel, S., Kumar, V.V., Rai, A., Eds.; Springer: Singapore, 2021. [CrossRef]
9. Boffano, P.; Roccia, F.; Gallesio, C.; Karagozoglu, K.H.; Forouzanfar, T. Diplopia and orbital wall fractures. *J. Craniofac. Surg.* **2014**, *25*, e183–e185. [CrossRef]
10. Boyette, J.R.; Pemberton, J.D.; Bonilla-Velez, J. Management of orbital fractures: Challenges and solutions. *Clin. Ophthalmol.* **2015**, *9*, 2127–2137. [CrossRef]
11. Ellis, E., 3rd; el-Attar, A.; Moos, K.F. An analysis of 2067 cases of zygomatic-orbital fracture. *J. Oral Maxillofac. Surg.* **1985**, *43*, 417–428. [CrossRef]
12. Nakamura, T.; Gross, C. Facial fractures: Analysis of five years of experience. *Arch. Otolaryngol.* **1973**, *97*, 288–290. [CrossRef] [PubMed]
13. Gwyn, P.P.; Carraway, J.H.; Horton, C.E. Facial fractures-injuries and associated complications. *Plast. Reconstr. Surg.* **1971**, *47*, 225–230. [CrossRef] [PubMed]
14. Miloro, M. *Peterson's Principles of Oral and Maxillofacial Surgery*; People's Medical Publishing House: Shelton, CT, USA, 2004.
15. Hauck, M.J.; Tao, J.P.; Burgett, R.A. Computed Tomography Exophthalmometry. *Ophthalmic Surg. Lasers Imaging Retina* **2010**, *22*, 1–4. [CrossRef] [PubMed]
16. Folkestad, L.; Lindgren, G.; Moller, C.; Granström, G. Diplopia in orbital fractures: A simple method to assess ocular motility. *Acta Otolaryngol.* **2007**, *127*, 156Y166. [CrossRef] [PubMed]
17. Timmis, P. Exophthalmos. *J. Laryngol. Otol.* **1957**, *71*, 744–753. [CrossRef] [PubMed]
18. Bartoli, D.; Fadda, M.T.; Battisti, A.; Cassoni, A.; Pagnoni, M.; Riccardi, E.; Sanzi, M.; Valentini, V. Retrospective analysis of 301 patients with orbital floor fracture. *J. Craniomaxillofac. Surg.* **2015**, *43*, 244–247. [CrossRef] [PubMed]
19. Hitchin, A.D.; Shuker, S.T. Some observations on zygomatic fractures in the Eastern Region of Scotland. *Br. J. Oral Surg.* **1973**, *11*, 114–117. [CrossRef]
20. Ramphul, A.; Hoffman, G. Does Preoperative Diplopia Determine the Incidence of Postoperative Diplopia After Repair of Orbital Floor Fracture? An Institutional Review. *J. Oral. Maxillofac. Surg.* **2017**, *75*, 565–575. [CrossRef]
21. Burm, J.S.; Chung, C.H.; Oh, S.J. Pure orbital blowout fracture: New concepts and importance of medial orbital blowout fracture. *Plast. Reconstr. Surg.* **1999**, *103*, 1839–1849. [CrossRef]
22. Higashino, T.; Hirabayashi, S.; Eguchi, T.; Kato, Y. Straightforward factors for predicting the prognosis of blow-out fractures. *J. Craniofac. Surg.* **2011**, *22*, 1210–1214. [CrossRef]
23. Eun, S.C.; Heo, C.Y.; Baek, R.M.; Minn, K.W.; Chung, C.H.; Oh, S.J. Survey and review of blowout fractures. *J. Korean Soc. Plast. Reconstr. Surg.* **2007**, *34*, 599–604.
24. Tahiri, Y.; Lee, J.; Tahiri, M.; Sinno, H.; Williams, B.H.; Lessard, L.; Gilardino, M.S. Preoperative diplopia: The most important prognostic factor for diplopia after surgical repair of pure orbital blowout fracture. *J. Craniofac. Surg.* **2010**, *21*, 1038–1041. [CrossRef] [PubMed]
25. Lee, K.M.; Park, J.U.; Kwon, S.T.; Kim, S.W.; Jeong, E.C. Three-dimensional pre-bent titanium implant for concomitant orbital floor and medial wall fractures in an East asian population. *Arch. Plast. Surg.* **2014**, *41*, 480–485. [CrossRef] [PubMed]
26. Thiagarajah, C.; Kersten, R.C. Medial wall fracture: An update. *Craniomaxillofac. Trauma Reconstr.* **2009**, *2*, 135–139. [CrossRef] [PubMed]
27. Kim, Y.H.; Park, Y.; Chung, K.J. Considerations for the management of medial orbital wall blowout fracture. *Arch. Plast. Surg.* **2016**, *43*, 229–236. [CrossRef]
28. Choi, S.H.; Kang, D.H.; Gu, J.H. The Correlation between the Orbital Volume Ratio and Enophthalmos in Unoperated Blowout Fractures. *Arch. Plast. Surg.* **2016**, *43*, 518–522. [CrossRef]
29. Bonavolontà, P.; Dell'aversana Orabona, G.; Abbate, V.; Vaira, L.A.; Lo Faro, C.; Petrocelli, M.; Attanasi, F.; De Riu, G.; Iaconetta, G.; Califano, L. The epidemiological analysis of maxillofacial fractures in Italy: The experience of a single tertiary center with 1720 patients. *J. Craniomaxillofac. Surg.* **2017**, *45*, 1319–1326. [CrossRef]
30. Orabona, G.D.; Abbate, V.; Maglitto, F.; Committeri, U.; Improta, G.; Bonavolontà, P.; Reccia, A.; Somma, T.; Iaconetta, G.; Califano, L. Postoperative Management of Zygomatic Arch Fractures: In-House Rapid Prototyping System for the Manufacture of Protective Facial Shields. *J. Craniofac. Surg.* **2019**, *30*, 2057–2060. [CrossRef]

Disclaimer/Publisher's Note: The statements, opinions and data contained in all publications are solely those of the individual author(s) and contributor(s) and not of MDPI and/or the editor(s). MDPI and/or the editor(s) disclaim responsibility for any injury to people or property resulting from any ideas, methods, instructions or products referred to in the content.

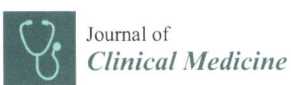

Article

Computed Tomography Morphology of Affected versus Unaffected Sides in Patients with Unilateral Primary Acquired Nasolacrimal Duct Obstruction

Pei-Yuan Su [1,2,*], Jia-Kang Wang [1] and Shu-Wen Chang [1]

1. Ophthalmology Department, Far-Eastern Memorial Hospital, New Taipei City 220, Taiwan
2. School of Medicine, Fu-Jen Catholic, New Taipei City 242062, Taiwan
* Correspondence: patsysu624@gmail.com; Tel.: +886-2-89667000 (ext. 1349)

Abstract: Background: This study aimed to describe the anatomical details of the bony nasolacrimal duct (BNLD) and adjacent nasal structures by analyzing computed tomography (CT) images, and to investigate their effects on the development of primary acquired nasolacrimal duct obstruction (PANDO). Methods: A total of 50 patients with unilateral PANDO who underwent dacryocystorhinostomy, with a mean age of 57.96 years, were included. The preoperative CT images were reviewed to measure the anteroposterior and transverse diameters of the BNLD at the entrance and exit levels, as well as the minimum transverse diameter along the tract. The sagittal CT images were analyzed to classify the shape of the bony canals into columnar, funnel, flare, and hourglass. The associated paranasal abnormalities, including nasal septum deviation (NSD), sinusitis, angle between the bony inferior turbinate and medial wall of the maxillary sinus, and mucosal thickness of the inferior turbinate, were investigated. Results: Fifty CT images were analyzed, and all parameters measured on both sides of the BNLD were not significantly different between the PANDO and non-PANDO sides, except for the minimum transverse diameter, which was significantly smaller on the PANDO side ($p = 0.002$). Columnar-shaped BNLD was the most common on both sides. No significant difference was observed in the incidence of paranasal abnormalities between sides; however, deviation of the septum toward the non-PANDO side was more common (67.9%). Conclusions: A small minimum transverse diameter of the BNLD may be a risk factor for PANDO. The association between nasal abnormalities and PANDO was not remarkable.

Keywords: primary acquired nasolacrimal duct obstruction; bony nasolacrimal duct; computed-tomography morphology

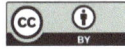

1. Introduction

Epiphora due to nasolacrimal duct obstruction (NLDO) is a common ophthalmic problem that accounts for approximately 3% of clinical visits [1]. The obstruction of the lacrimal drainage system can be congenital or acquired. Congenital NLDO, which presents symptoms soon after birth, commonly results from a persistent membrane at the valve of Hasner. Acquired NLDO, which manifests later in life, can be classified into primary or secondary NLDO. Common causes of secondary acquired NLDO include facial trauma or surgery, neoplasm, sarcoidosis, and Wegener's granulomatosis [2].

Primary acquired NLDO (PANDO) is frequent among older women and is usually bilateral. PANDO is characterized by gradual chronic inflammation and fibrosis along the nasolacrimal duct, leading to obstruction of the drainage system [1,3]. Although PANDO is idiopathic, many predisposing factors, such as conjunctival infection, nasal disease, hormone fluctuation, sinusitis, female sex, smoking, and topical glaucoma medication, have been suggested [1,4–6].

Anatomical variation of the bony nasolacrimal duct (BNLD) is also a crucial risk factor for PANDO. Narrowing of the bony canal may cause stasis of the tear flow, accumulation of debris and inflammatory products, adhesion and fibrosis of the internal nasolacrimal duct mucosa, and finally obstruction of the drainage pathway. Some studies have compared the diameter of the BNLD among normal individuals of different age groups, sexes, and ethnicities [7–9]. One study reported a smaller diameter of the BNLD in the PANDO group than in the control group; however, other studies have reported no significant difference in the BNLD diameter between the groups [7,10–13]. Therefore, the results on the role of BNLD morphology in the development of PANDO are controversial. Because of the anatomical proximity, the lacrimal drainage pathway may be affected by pathology in the nasal cavity and paranasal sinuses [14]. Relationships between PANDO and paranasal sinusitis, nasal septum deviation (NSD), the angle between the bony inferior turbinate and nasal lateral wall at the end of the nasolacrimal duct, and structural abnormalities of the sinonasal cavity have been studied [15–18]; however, the results are inconclusive.

To determine the risk factors for PANDO, we compared the morphology of the BNLD and sinonasal abnormality of the affected (PANDO) and unaffected (non-PANDO) sides of our patients with unilateral PANDO by reviewing computed tomography (CT) images. Observations included the bony canal diameter at different levels, aeration inside the canal, the canal shape in sagittal view, NSD severity, the presence of sinusitis, and inferior turbinate structure at the distal end of the BNLD.

2. Materials and Methods

2.1. Participants and Ethics

This study was approved by the Institutional Review Board of Far Eastern Memorial Hospital, New Taipei City, Taiwan (NO. 111038-E), and the tenets of the Declaration of Helsinki were followed. The preoperative orbital CT scans of all patients with unilateral PANDO who presented to our ophthalmology clinic from December 2019 to May 2021 were retrospectively reviewed. The diagnosis of PANDO was made through lacrimal irrigation and probing under topical anesthesia in the outpatient department. Once the patients agreed to receive further surgical intervention, orbital CT scans were obtained to rule out lacrimal sac tumors or nasal pathologies that could cause secondary NLDO. Patients with congenital NLDO; bilateral PANDO; NLDO secondary to trauma, tumor, or orbital irradiation; or a history of sinusitis or lacrimal surgery were excluded. A total of 50 patients with unilateral PANDO were included, and CT scan images of the PANDO and non-PANDO sides were evaluated separately.

2.2. Data Retrieval and Processing

CT scans were performed using a 64-slice high-speed scanner (SOMATOM Definition AS; Siemens, Munich, Germany). Contiguous 2 mm axial and sagittal images were obtained parallel and perpendicular to the orbital floor. Anatomical measurements were made by a single investigator by using the caliber tools of the viewer through bone windows.

To evaluate BNLD morphology, the anteroposterior and transverse diameters of the inner bony canal in axial view were measured at three levels: the entrance point at the inferior orbital margin, the exit point at the opening of the inferior meatus, and the minimum transverse diameter along the bony canal (Figure 1). In the sagittal view, the longest section of the BNLD, in which proximal and distal ends were visible, was selected for evaluating the shape of the bony canal. We classified the BNLD shape into four types according to the location of the narrow point (the minimum anteroposterior diameter) within the bony canal (Figure 2). In the funnel type, the narrow point was located near the exit level of the BNLD, whereas in the flare type, the narrow point was located at the BNLD entrance. In the hourglass type, the narrow point was located between the exit and entrance levels. In the columnar type, the anteroposterior diameters of the inner BNLD were evenly distributed along the pathway.

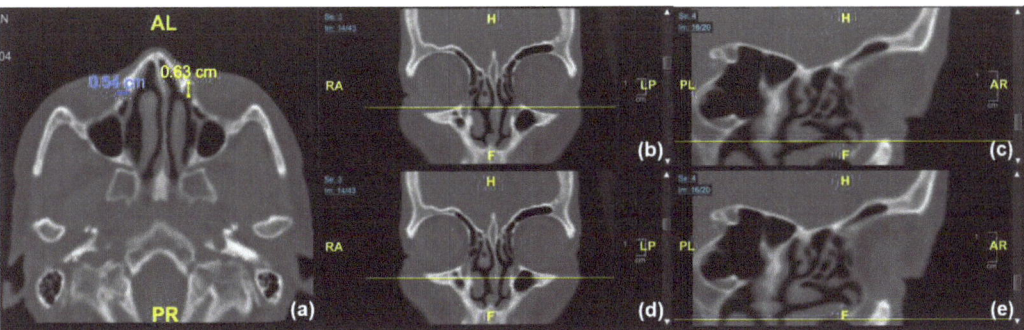

Figure 1. (**a**) Anteroposterior and transverse diameters of the inner bony canal in axial view. The diameters were measured at three levels: the entrance point at inferior orbital margin (**b**,**c**), the exit point at the opening of inferior meatus (**d**,**e**), and the minimum transverse diameter along the bony canal.

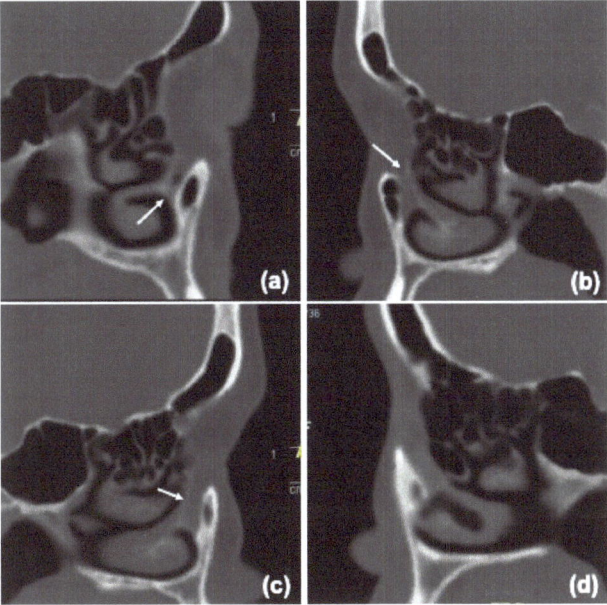

Figure 2. Four shapes of the BNLD. (**a**) Funnel type: narrow point near the exit level. (**b**) Flare type: narrow point near the entrance level. (**c**) Hourglass type: narrow point between the exit and entrance levels. (**d**) Columnar type: evenly distributed along the path.

To evaluate the anatomy of the part of the nasal cavity into which the nasolacrimal duct drained, a single coronal section of the CT image corresponding to the most distal part of the BNLD was selected. Measurements included the NSD angle, the angle between the bony inferior turbinate and medial wall of the maxillary sinus, and transverse mucosal thickness of the inferior turbinate (Figure 3). The NSD angle was measured by drawing a vertical line from the crista galli to the nasal crest of the maxillary bone and another line to the maximum deviation of the nasal septum.

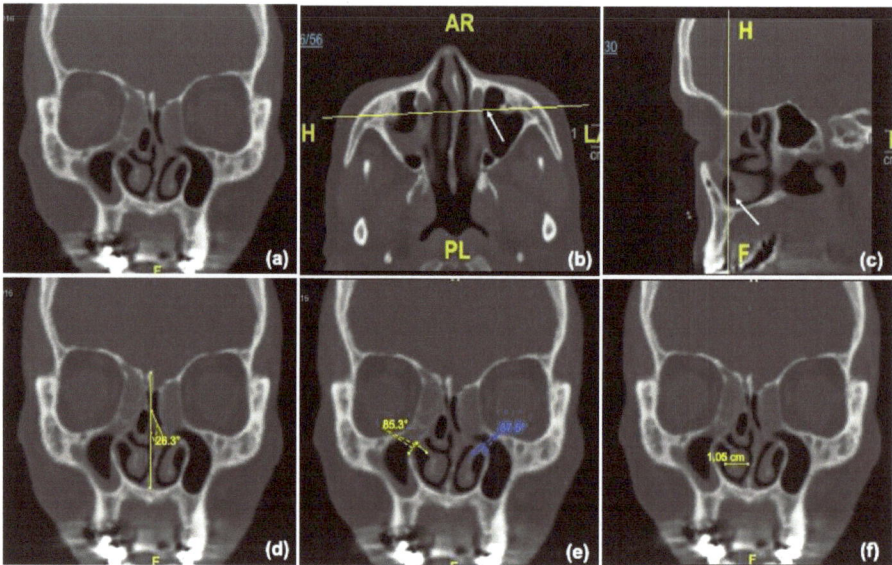

Figure 3. (**a**) Coronal sections corresponding to the most distal part of the BNLD were selected (**b**) from axial and (**c**) sagittal CT images. Measurements included NSD angle (**d**), angle between the bony inferior turbinate and medial wall of the maxillary sinus (**e**), and transverse mucosal thickness of the inferior turbinate (**f**).

2.3. Statistical Analyses

Statistical analyses were performed using SPSS 23.0. The independent sample t test, chi-squared test, and Pearson's correlation were used. A p value of <0.05 was considered statistically significant.

3. Results

Patient Characteristics and Measurement Results

A total of 50 patients with unilateral PANDO (4 men and 46 women) and a mean age of 57.96 years (ranging from 35 to 77 years) were included. PANDO laterality was equally distributed among the patients (25 left and 25 right sides).

The BNLD measurement results of the PANDO and non-PANDO sides are listed in Table 1. The mean anteroposterior diameter and transverse diameter of both sides were not significantly different over the entrance level (p = 0.439 and 0.188, respectively). No significant differences in the mean anteroposterior diameter and transverse diameter were observed between the sides at the exit level (p = 0.357 and 0.085, respectively). However, significantly smaller minimum transverse diameters were observed on the PANDO sides (mean ± SD = 3.63 ± 1.08 mm) than on the non-PANDO sides (mean ± SD = 4.07 ± 1.13 mm; p = 0.002), and same results were obtained for both sexes (p = 0.016 for female and 0.023 for male). We also found that mean minimum transverse diameters were significantly larger in males on both sides (p = 0.014 on PANDO sides and 0.036 on non-PANDO sides. Comparisons of the BNLD measurements between sexes are summarized in Table 2. All measured parameters were not correlated with age for either the PANDO or non-PANDO sides; the results are summarized in Table 3.

Table 1. Measurements of the bony nasolacrimal duct.

	PANDO Side		Non-PANDO Side		p-Value	
	A-P Diameter	Transverse Diameter	A-P Diameter	Transverse Diameter		
	Mean ± SD (mm)					
Entrance	5.77 ± 1.39	4.49 ± 1.32	5.76 ± 1.30	4.58 ± 1.31	0.439	0.188
Exit	7.06 ± 1.94	4.22 ± 1.15	7.00 ± 1.79	4.37 ± 1.05	0.357	0.085
Minimum		3.63 ± 1.08		4.07 ± 1.13		0.002 *

PANDO: primary acquired nasolacrimal duct obstruction; A-P: Anteroposterior; * Statistically significant according to independent *t* test.

Table 2. Comparison of the bony nasolacrimal duct between sexes.

	PANDO Side		Non-PANDO Side		p-Value	
Diameter	A-P	Transverse	A-P	Transverse		
	Mean ± SD (mm)		Mean ± SD (mm)			
Female (n = 46)						
Entrance	5.77 ± 1.39	4.37 ± 1.24	5.73 ± 1.29	4.46 ± 1.24	0.444	0.353
Exit	7.03 ± 2.01	4.19 ± 1.19	6.90 ± 1.78	4.27 ± 1.01	0.263	0.076
Minimum		3.57 ± 1.08		3.98 ± 1.11		0.016 *
Male (n = 4)						
Entrance	5.83 ± 1.62	5.95 ± 1.51	6.10 ± 1.51	5.93 ± 1.44	0.406	0.491
Exit	7.38 ± 0.85	4.60 ± 0.39	8.08 ± 1.65	5.48 ± 0.92	0.240	0.066
Minimum		4.70 ± 0.55		5.10 ± 0.85		0.023 *
p-value						
Entrance	0.474	0.062	0.331	0.066		
Exit	0.263	0.076	0.127	0.073		
Minimum		0.014 **		0.036 **		

PANDO: primary acquired nasolacrimal duct obstruction; A-P: Anteroposterior; * Statistically significant according to independent *t* test; ** Statistically significant according Mann–Whitney U test.

Table 3. Correlation between age and the bony nasolacrimal duct.

	Entrance Level		Minimum Transverse Diameter	Exit Level	
	A-P Diameter	Transverse Diameter		A-P Diameter	Transverse Diameter
			r (correlation coefficient)		
PANDO side	0.170	0.202	0.179	0.194	0.057
non-PANDO side	0.273	0.225	0.205	0.211	0.206

PANDO: primary acquired nasolacrimal duct obstruction; A-P: Anteroposterior; r: Pearson's correlation coefficient.

The analysis of the BNDL shape using sagittal CT images of the orbits revealed that the most common shape of the BNLD was columnar (accounting for 48% and 66% of the PANDO and non-PANDO sides, respectively), followed by flare, funnel, and hourglass. No significant difference in the BNLD shape was observed between the PANDO and non-PANDO sides ($p = 0.205$); the results are listed in Table 4.

Table 4. Shape of the bony nasolacrimal duct.

	PANDO Side		Non-PANDO Side	
	n	(%)	n	(%)
Columnar	24	48	33	66
Flare	17	34	11	22
Funnel	4	8	2	4
Hourglass	5	10	4	8

PANDO: primary acquired nasolacrimal duct obstruction.

The CT images revealed that 28 patients (56%) had NSD, with a mean angle of deviation of 5.38° ± 6.38° (ranging from 3.2° to 26.3°). Of them, 19 patients (67.9%) had their septum deviated to the non-PANDO side. The measurements of the coronal section corresponding to the exit level of the BNLD revealed that the mean angle between the bony inferior turbinate and medial wall of the maxillary sinus was 53.84° ± 17.94° on the PANDO sides and 54.73° ± 15.38° on the non-PANDO sides. No significant difference in the mean angle was observed between the sides ($p = 0.295$). The mean highest transverse mucosal thickness of the inferior turbinate from the same coronal section was 8.47 ± 1.60 mm on the PANDO sides and 8.25 ± 1.97 mm on the non-PANDO sides. No significant difference in the mean highest transverse mucosal thickness was observed between the sides ($p = 0.196$). The CT images revealed that 10 patients (20%) had an opacity of the paranasal sinus on the PANDO sides, whereas 7 patients (14%) had an opacity of the paranasal sinus on the non-PANDO sides. No significant difference in opacity was observed between the sides ($p = 0.323$).

4. Discussion

Several studies have measured the BNLD diameter in the normal population. By measuring the epoxy resin casts of macerated skulls, Steinkogler [3] reported a transverse BNLD diameter of 4.8 mm. Janssen [7] included 100 controls in a study in the Netherlands and determined the mean minimum transverse diameter to be 3.7 mm in men and 3.35 mm in women by reviewing axial CT images. Lee [8] reported a mean transverse diameter of 4.5 mm and a minimum transverse diameter of 3.2 mm among 228 Korean patients without NLDO. Takahashi [12] reviewed the CT images of 100 sides of 50 Japanese patients without NLDO and reported a minimum transverse diameter of 4.8 mm. Fasina [11] measured the minimum BNLD diameter of 401 Nigerian adults using CT images and reported a diameter of 3.52 mm in men and 3.36 mm in women. In our study of Taiwanese adults, the minimum transverse diameter was 4.07 mm on the non-PANDO sides, which was higher than those in the aforementioned study groups except for the Takahashi group's results for the Japanese population. Although the prevalence of PANDO is lower among Africans than among Caucasians and Asians, the impact of ethnicity on PANDO is not conclusive from the perspective of BNLD size.

A small diameter of the bony canal is one of the proposed etiological factors contributing to NLDO. One study calculated the flow resistance in a tube by using an equation and reported that a 0.3 mm reduction in tube diameter increases resistance to the water flow by 1.38 times [9]. In our study, the anteroposterior and transverse diameters of the BNLD were not significantly different between the PANDO and non-PANDO sides at either the entrance or exit levels. However, the minimum transverse diameter on the PANDO sides (3.63 ± 1.08 mm) was significantly smaller than that on the non-PANDO sides (4.07 ± 1.13 mm; $p = 0.002$), and the difference was more than 0.3 mm. Similar results were reported by Janssen et al. [7], wherein the minimum transverse diameter of the BNLD was smaller in patients with PANDO than in controls (3.0 vs. 3.5 mm, $p = 0.001$). However, the sample size of the study was small (the patient group $n = 24$, the control group $n = 100$). Another comparative study by Takahashi [12] with a larger sample size (101 patients with unilateral PANDO and 50 controls) reported that the minimum transverse diameter on the NLDO sides was 5.09 mm, that on non-NLDO sides was 4.96 mm, and that on control sides was 4.80 mm. However, no significant difference in the minimum transverse diameter was noted between the groups. Bulbul [13] enrolled 39 patients with unilateral PANDO and 36 controls and discovered that the minimum and distal transverse diameters of the BNLD in patients with PANDO were significantly smaller than those in controls ($p = 0.04$ and <0.001, respectively). However, no differences in any BNLD measurements were observed between the NLDO and non-NLDO sides in patients with PANDO. The results of previous studies varied. Though the possibility of future development of nasolacrimal duct obstruction in the presently unaffected eyes cannot be ruled out, our results suggest that eyes with smaller BNLD diameter are prone to early presence of PANDO.

Changes in the lumen along the lacrimal passage may also influence the resistance of the tear flow [8]. Takahashi [12] reported that funnel-shaped BNLD with a minimum diameter at the canal entrance was more common in patients with NLDO than in controls. Moreover, because funnel-shaped BNLD was more common among female patients with NLDO, they concluded that this shape may increase the incidence of NLDO among women.

To evaluate the effect of different narrow-point locations on the formation of an obstruction, we described the shapes of the BNLD and classified them into four types, columnar, flare, funnel, and hourglass. Our study demonstrated that columnar-shaped BNLD was the most common on both PANDO and non-PANDO sides. Though the results showed that there was no statistically significant difference in proportion for all types between the two sides, we did find that noncolumnar types were more frequently observed on PANDO sides compared to non-PANDO sides (52% vs. 34%). Few studies have emphasized the relationship of the BNLD shape or location of the narrow point with NLDO occurrence. Our study provides a more detailed description of the canal shape according to location of narrowing, and supports the idea that changes in canal size along the tract despite different levels might play a role in the etiology of PANDO. Further studies should be conducted to compare these results with those of the normal population.

The relationship between the occurrence of PANDO and paranasal sinus pathology remains controversial. Kallman [19] evaluated the CT images of 23 patients with PANDO and 100 controls and reported a significantly higher rate of abnormal paranasal sinus findings, including NSD and ethmoidal opacification, in the PANDO group (87% vs. 63%). Dikici [18] investigated the CT images of 37 patients with PANDO and 37 controls and discovered a significant relationship between PANDO and axial location or NSD angle. Habesoglu [17] studied 41 patients with unilateral PANDO and reported no significant difference in the rates of NSD and ethmoidal sinusitis between the PANDO and control groups. Yazici [15] compared 40 unilateral PANDO patients with 71 controls and discovered no significant difference in the incidence of paranasal sinus abnormalities, including NSD location, NSD angle, and sinusitis, between the PANDO sides and the non-PANDO sides or controls. A correlation was observed only between the NSD and PANDO sides. Our study revealed that 56% of the patients with unilateral PANDO had NSD. Moreover, the nasal septum deviated more toward the non-PANDO sides (67.9%), a result contradictory to that of Yazici's study. However, the incidence of paranasal sinusitis in our study was not significantly different between the PANDO and non-PANDO sides ($p = 0.323$). The varying results may be due to the lack of a standard definition for all paranasal sinus pathologies, such as NSD location or sinusitis severity. Previous studies have demonstrated that NSD is one of the common causes of dacryocystorhinostomy failure [20,21], which may be attributed to the obstruction of surgical access or postoperative adhesion leading to ostium closure. The role of NSD in the development of PANDO remains inconclusive.

Narrowing of the nasal structure at the distal opening of the nasolacrimal duct is considered a predisposing factor for the occurrence of PANDO. Yazici [15] discovered no difference in mucosal thickness and the lateralization angle of the inferior turbinate between the NLDO and non-NLDO groups. Gul [16] reported that the mean angle between the bony inferior turbinate and medial wall of the maxillary sinus was significantly narrower on the affected sides than on the unaffected sides in the PANDO group (56.2° vs. 58.6°, $p = 0.01$). Dikici [18] compared the angle width between the bony inferior turbinate and medial wall of the maxillary sinus between patients with PANDO and controls and discovered that the angle was significantly wider on both sides in patients with PANDO ($p = 0.007$ for the right sides and $p = 0.006$ for the left sides). In our study, no significant difference in either the mucosal thickness of the inferior turbinate or angle between the bony inferior turbinate and medial wall of the maxillary sinus was observed between the PANDO and non-PANDO sides ($p = 0.295$ and 0.196, respectively). The nasolacrimal duct opens into the vault of the meatus located underneath the inferior turbinate, but it may extend further down and open at various positions in nasal lateral wall. Therefore, we speculated that the location selected for the measurement of the inferior turbinate angle width may not truly reflect the impact of the narrow nasal structure on the drainage of tear duct.

Our study was limited by the retrospective study design and the lack of a normal control group for comparison. Moreover, the possibility of PANDO development on unaffected sides in the future cannot be ruled out. Future studies using three-dimensional

CT image reconstruction may be needed to demonstrate the details of the bony structure of nasolacrimal duct more precisely.

5. Conclusions

In conclusion, columnar-shaped BNLD, with no obvious narrowing along the path on either side, was more frequent among our patients with unilateral PANDO. A smaller minimum transverse diameter of the bony canal was observed on the PANDO sides than on the non-PANDO sides, which might indicate a risk factor for NLDO. The nasal septum deviated more toward the non-PANDO sides. No significant difference in the lateralization of the bony inferior turbinate, mucosal thickness of the inferior turbinate, or incidence of sinusitis was observed between the sides. The association between nasal abnormalities and NLDO remains unclear. Our study provides information on anatomical details of the BNLD and associated nasal structures, thereby improving the understanding of PANDO pathophysiology.

Author Contributions: Conceptualization, J.-K.W., S.-W.C. and P.-Y.S.; methodology, J.-K.W., S.-W.C. and P.-Y.S.; software, P.-Y.S.; validation, J.-K.W., S.-W.C. and P.-Y.S.; formal analysis, P.-Y.S.; investigation, P.-Y.S.; resources, J.-K.W., S.-W.C. and P.-Y.S.; data curation, P.-Y.S.; writing—original draft preparation, P.-Y.S.; writing—review and editing, P.-Y.S.; visualization, J.-K.W., S.-W.C. and P.-Y.S.; supervision, J.-K.W. and S.-W.C.; project administration, P.-Y.S. All authors have read and agreed to the published version of the manuscript.

Funding: This research received no external funding.

Institutional Review Board Statement: The study was conducted according to the guidelines of the Declaration of Helsinki and approved by the Institutional Review Board of Far-Eastern Memorial Hospital (NO. 111038-E, approval by 14 March 2022).

Informed Consent Statement: Patient consent was waived as all subjects had completed their treatment before they were included, and their clinical treatment would not be affected by the study. Throughout the data processing, identifiable information was removed and kept strictly confidential.

Data Availability Statement: Not applied.

Acknowledgments: The authors would like to express our thanks to the staff of the Far-Eastern Memorial Hospital Statistical Consulting Unit for statistical consultation and analyses.

Conflicts of Interest: The authors declare no conflict of interest.

References

1. Linberg, J.V.; McCormick, S.A. Primary acquired nasolacrimal duct obstruction. A clinicopathologic report and biopsy technique. *Ophthalmology* **1986**, *93*, 1055–1063. [CrossRef]
2. Bartley, G.B. Acquired lacrimal drainage obstruction: An etiologic classification system, case reports, and a review of the literature. Part 3. *Ophthalmic Plast Reconstr. Surg.* **1993**, *9*, 11–26. [CrossRef] [PubMed]
3. Steinkogler, F.J. The postsaccal, idiopathic dacryostenosis—Experimental and clinical aspects. *Doc. Ophthalmol.* **1986**, *63*, 265–286. [CrossRef] [PubMed]
4. Kashkouli, M.B.; Sadeghipour, A.; Kaghazkanani, R.; Bayat, A.; Pakdel, F.; Aghai, G.H. Pathogenesis of primary acquired nasolacrimal duct obstruction. *Orbit* **2010**, *29*, 11–15. [CrossRef] [PubMed]
5. Ohtomo, K.; Ueta, T.; Toyama, T.; Nagahara, M. Predisposing factors for primary acquired nasolacrimal duct obstruction. *Graefes Arch. Clin. Exp. Ophthalmol.* **2013**, *251*, 1835–1839. [CrossRef] [PubMed]
6. Seider, N.; Miller, B.; Beiran, I. Topical glaucoma therapy as a risk factor for nasolacrimal duct obstruction. *Am. J. Ophthalmol.* **2008**, *145*, 120–123. [CrossRef] [PubMed]
7. Janssen, A.G.; Mansour, K.; Bos, J.J.; Castelijns, J.A. Diameter of the bony lacrimal canal: Normal values and values related to nasolacrimal duct obstruction: Assessment with CT. *AJNR Am. J. Neuroradiol.* **2001**, *22*, 845–850. [PubMed]
8. Lee, H.; Ha, S.; Lee, Y.; Park, M.; Baek, S. Anatomical and morphometric study of the bony nasolacrimal canal using computed tomography. *Ophthalmologica* **2012**, *227*, 153–159. [CrossRef]
9. McCormick, A.; Sloan, B. The diameter of the nasolacrimal canal measured by computed tomography: Gender and racial differences. *Clin. Exp. Ophthalmol.* **2009**, *37*, 357–361. [CrossRef]
10. Takahashi, Y.; Nakamura, Y.; Nakano, T.; Asamoto, K.; Iwaki, M.; Selva, D.; Leibovitch, I.; Kakizaki, H. The narrowest part of the bony nasolacrimal canal: An anatomical study. *Ophthalmic Plast. Reconstr. Surg.* **2013**, *29*, 318–322. [CrossRef]

11. Fasina, O.; Ogbole, G.I. CT assessment of the nasolacrimal canal in a black African Population. *Ophthalmic Plast Reconstr. Surg.* **2013**, *29*, 231–233. [CrossRef] [PubMed]
12. Takahashi, Y.; Nakata, K.; Miyazaki, H.; Ichinose, A.; Kakizaki, H. Comparison of bony nasolacrimal canal narrowing with or without primary acquired nasolacrimal duct obstruction in a Japanese population. *Ophthalmic Plast Reconstr. Surg.* **2014**, *30*, 434–438. [CrossRef] [PubMed]
13. Bulbul, E.; Yazici, A.; Yanik, B.; Yazici, H.; Demirpolat, G. Morphometric Evaluation of Bony Nasolacrimal Canal in a Caucasian Population with Primary Acquired Nasolacrimal Duct Obstruction: A Multidetector Computed Tomography Study. *Korean J. Radiol.* **2016**, *17*, 271–276. [CrossRef] [PubMed]
14. Ali, M.J.; Paulsen, F. Etiopathogenesis of Primary Acquired Nasolacrimal Duct Obstruction: What We Know and What We Need to Know. *Ophthalmic Plast Reconstr. Surg.* **2019**, *35*, 426–433. [CrossRef] [PubMed]
15. Yazici, H.; Bulbul, E.; Yazici, A.; Kaymakci, M.; Tiskaoglu, N.; Yanik, B.; Ermis, S. Primary acquired nasolacrimal duct obstruction: Is it really related to paranasal abnormalities? *Surg. Radiol. Anat.* **2015**, *37*, 579–584. [CrossRef]
16. Gul, A.; Aslan, K.; Karli, R.; Ariturk, N.; Can, E. A Possible Cause of Nasolacrimal Duct Obstruction: Narrow Angle between Inferior Turbinate and Upper Part of the Medial Wall of the Maxillary Sinus. *Curr. Eye Res.* **2016**, *41*, 729–733. [CrossRef] [PubMed]
17. Habesoglu, M.; Eriman, M.; Habesoglu, T.E.; Kinis, V.; Surmeli, M.; Deveci, I.; Deveci, S. Co-occurrence and possible role of sinonasal anomalies in primary acquired nasolacrimal duct obstruction. *J. Craniofac. Surg.* **2013**, *24*, 497–500. [CrossRef]
18. Dikici, O.; Ulutas, H.G. Relationship between Primary Acquired Nasolacrimal Duct Obstruction, Paranasal Abnormalities and Nasal Septal Deviation. *J. Craniofac. Surg.* **2020**, *31*, 782–786. [CrossRef]
19. Kallman, J.E.; Foster, J.A.; Wulc, A.E.; Yousem, D.M.; Kennedy, D.W. Computed tomography in lacrimal outflow obstruction. *Ophthalmology* **1997**, *104*, 676–682. [CrossRef]
20. Dalgic, A.; Ceylan, M.E.; Celik, C.; Aliyeva, A.; Aksoy, G.Y.; Edizer, D.T. Outcomes of Endoscopic Powered Revision Dacryocystorhinostomy. *J. Craniofac. Surg.* **2018**, *29*, 1960–1962. [CrossRef]
21. Lin, G.C.; Brook, C.D.; Hatton, M.P.; Metson, R. Causes of dacryocystorhinostomy failure: External versus endoscopic approach. *Am. J. Rhinol. Allergy* **2017**, *31*, 181–185. [CrossRef] [PubMed]

Disclaimer/Publisher's Note: The statements, opinions and data contained in all publications are solely those of the individual author(s) and contributor(s) and not of MDPI and/or the editor(s). MDPI and/or the editor(s) disclaim responsibility for any injury to people or property resulting from any ideas, methods, instructions or products referred to in the content.

MDPI AG
Grosspeteranlage 5
4052 Basel
Switzerland
Tel.: +41 61 683 77 34

Journal of Clinical Medicine Editorial Office
E-mail: jcm@mdpi.com
www.mdpi.com/journal/jcm

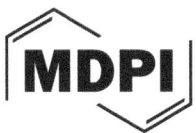

Disclaimer/Publisher's Note: The title and front matter of this reprint are at the discretion of the Guest Editors. The publisher is not responsible for their content or any associated concerns. The statements, opinions and data contained in all individual articles are solely those of the individual Editors and contributors and not of MDPI. MDPI disclaims responsibility for any injury to people or property resulting from any ideas, methods, instructions or products referred to in the content.

www.ingramcontent.com/pod-product-compliance
Lightning Source LLC
LaVergne TN
LVHW070003100526
838202LV00019B/2614